THE
OFFICIAL
CAMBRIDGE
DIET BOOK

To Aldie + Ira —
who are
infuriatingly never
in need of
any diet.

LOVE!
Rene Boe

THE
OFFICIAL
CAMBRIDGE
DIET BOOK

by
Eugene Boe

BANTAM BOOKS
TORONTO · NEW YORK · LONDON · SYDNEY

THE OFFICIAL CAMBRIDGE DIET BOOK
A Bantam Book / April 1983

All rights reserved.
Copyright © 1983 by Eugene Boe.
Designed by Gene Siegel
This book may not be reproduced in whole or in part, by mimeograph or
any other means, without permission.
For information address: Bantam Books, Inc.

ISBN 0-553-34025-5

Published simultaneously in the United States and Canada

PRINTED IN THE UNITED STATES OF AMERICA

CW   0 9 8 7 6 5 4 3 2 1

CONTENTS

INTRODUCTION

Prior to the formulations of the Cambridge Diet, I had spent almost twenty years in obesity research. My consuming interest was to discover a safe, efficient means of achieving weight reduction and thereby come to grips with a major health hazard that affects millions of people throughout the world.

At the beginning of my investigations, the most popular treatment among physicians was complete starvation — the zero-calorie diet. Besides being extremely hazardous, it had to be restricted to the relatively few people who could be institutionalized and kept under careful scrutiny.

My first objective was to learn the minimum amounts of macro-nutrients and calories needed by overweight people on a weight-loss diet, with the aim of achieving the fastest possible weight loss with maximum safety. Having arrived at that formula, my medical colleagues and I had to test it thoroughly on hundreds of patients, to substantiate and confirm that it was indeed safe.

Nothing has been more gratifying to me — and the many doctors and scientists who have worked with me — than the astonishing acceptability of what has become known as the Cambridge Diet. By good fortune and much endeavour, we developed a diet that millions of people appear to like and can stay with. It achieves what we sought — a dramatic and speedy weight loss, while at the same time increasing energy and enhancing good health and nutrition.

Alan N. Howard, Ph.D., F.R.I.C.

1

THE CAMBRIDGE DIET—
REVOLUTIONARY!

 Why is the Cambridge Diet different from all other diets? *Better* than all other diets? Why is it unique, and why is it sweeping the country with a fervor unsurpassed by any other diet *ever*?

The answer is simple: The Cambridge Diet works!

- It is the fastest *safe* way to dramatic weight loss.
- It is the truly "educated" diet—a result of nearly a decade of research and clinical testing by scientists and physicians at the University of Cambridge, in English hospitals, and by research teams throughout Europe. *No other diet has ever been so thoroughly tested for safety, effectiveness, and acceptability.*
- It is a very low calorie diet—and the *only* very low calorie diet available to the public that contains the known vital nutrients the body requires for short periods and has them aligned in perfect balance.
- It is *not* a fad diet. Fad diets are unbalanced, omitting essential nutrients or having too much of something.

- It is simplicity itself. It takes only minutes to prepare — "the ultimate in futuristic fast food", according to *Harper's Bazaar*.
- It is natural. It contains no drugs, stimulants, medication, or preservatives of any kind.
- It significantly lowers serum cholesterol and triglyceride levels.
- It has a low sodium content — an added blessing for people with high blood pressure.
- It is easy to live with. Its concentration of nutrients squelches hunger sensations.
- It has no serious side effects.
- It has versatility.
- It is highly palatable.
- Its sources of protein — soy flour, nonfat dry milk solids, and hydrolized vegetable protein — also make it a boon to vegetarians.
- It provides the dieter with a concerned network of supervision and mutual support, the Cambridge Counselors.
- It is the answer to the problem of lifetime weight maintenance.
- It is inexpensive: one meal costs less than a dollar.
- It is patented — the truest testimonial to its uniqueness.

The Cambridge Diet is the gateway to a whole new life — a life that is richer, healthier, happier, and more energized than the one that was shed with the excess poundage.

2

THE EXTENDED FAMILY
OF CAMBRIDGE

"The Cambridge Obsession," a trendy magazine dubbed it. "A new diet has attracted hysterical devotion..."

"Absolutely *everybody's* on it, darling," trills one of the more vivacious darlings of New York's Disco Society.

Well, not *everybody's* on it. Not yet.

But the diet that came onto the market scarcely three years ago has already beat a pathway to the door of millions.

To the Cambridge Diet have come the likes of royalty, entertainers, athletes, politicians, writers, columnists, cartoonists, doctors, and lots and lots of everybody else.

Yes!

Even a member of the British Royal Family has found the way to Cambridge.

So have some of the biggest names in Hollywood, the hottest Country and Western singers, blazing comets of the rock galaxy, talk show hosts,

3

wild comics, Miss Americas and Playmates of the Year, Las Vegas spellbinders, songwriters and D.J.'s, Metropolitan Opera mezzo sopranos and baritones, and the whole constellation of powers that surround and nurture and present and represent these talents.

"I hear Cambridge *everywhere*", exclaims the beautiful promotion chief of a cosmetics dynasty. "I walk down the hall and I literally see people *melting* before my eyes."

Cambridge is the sporting way, to say the least.

Many sports figures have discovered Cambridge!

Supernovas of the National Football League, the National Basketball Association, the National and American (baseball) Leagues, and the National Hockey League are rapturous converts. Likewise their managers and trainers and coaches. Likewise a World Heavyweight Champion boxer. Likewise World Champion ice skaters and Olympic champs.

Our nation's capital has taken to Cambridge with a passion. "You wouldn't believe some of the names who are reaching out for the Cambridge Diet as if it were Nirvana", gushes a Washington columnist. Well, yes you would. Particularly if you had been watching a famous senator — a gentleman who is by no means allergic to the limelight — *shrinking* on network television news night after night.

Physicans in increasing numbers are proclaiming the powerhouse of the Cambridge Diet. And backing up their proclamations by putting themselves on it and recommending it to their patients.

Count also among Cambridge users some three million other stars — your neighbors and mine!

3

THIN IS IN: FAT IS OUT, UGLY, AND DANGEROUS

Doctors, even those who are overweight themselves, advise us, "You'd better go on a diet."

Public officials warn that being overweight is the number one health problem in the country. With every excess pound we are measurably increasing the chances of ending our days prematurely.

As the U.S. Public Health Service declared in its 1979 National Institute of Health publication *Obesity in America*: "It can be estimated...that if everyone were at optimal weight, we would have 25 percent less coronary heart disease and 35 percent less congestive failure and brain infarctions. This potential benefit seems worth considerable effort to control or, better yet, to avoid obesity."

"We are digging our graves with our teeth," nutritionists intone.

If we do not die of the likely consequences of overeating—heart attacks, strokes, diabetes, general poor health—we risk being nagged to death about our gluttonous habits.

Between 70 and 80 million of us are overweight, despite the fact that our society attaches a powerful stigma to being fat.

Psychologists tell us obesity enjoys about the same amount of general esteem as drug addiction. Overweight people are perceived as individuals who have let themselves go, who could correct their condition if they chose to. They are seen as unhealthy, undisciplined, unattractive, and unstable. Part of the stigma of fat is that fat is not associated with success.

Thus, we have become a nation of dieters.

Approximately every other American considers himself overweight. This year about four out of ten Americans will go on some sort of diet.

At this very moment at least 20 million of us are "seriously dieting."

In 1982 we spent about $200 million on weight-loss preparations and diet books.

A 1981 National Center for Health Statistics survey found that 58 percent of all Americans are more than five percent over their desired weight, and 15 percent are overweight by *at least* 30 percent. "With advancing age," states the study, "there is a small but steady decline in the proportion of persons reporting optimal weight."

A sizeable segment of us feel that we eat too much of the "wrong" foods — snacks, sweets, starches and fat.

We *are* diet oriented.

This penchant for dieting seems to be related to our notions about what the "good life" should be in terms of health and social acceptance.

We are, as people, health conscious and quick to recognize all the advantages of being physically fit.

A recent Gallup poll disclosed that Americans ranked good physical health second only to good family life.

And yet, with all this talk about good nutrition and proper weight, we have only to look around us to see that good intentions are too rarely translated into action.

Present economic difficulties notwithstanding, this is still the richest country in the world. It is still within the means of the vast majority of us to be sensibly well-fed. But only three out of ten people, according to a Hoffman-La Roche investigation, consider themselves to be in excellent nutritional shape. Only about half the people could even identify the basic food groups essential to a good diet.

There are encouraging signs. "We are what we eat," we openly acknowledge. More and more people are calorie conscious; they are reading labels on food and beverage products for ingredient information.

The term "junk foods" has entered into the common parlance. Increasingly, many of us are turning away from salt-and-sugar loaded foods, cutting down on our consumption of fried foods, high-fat dairy products, red meat, and hard liquor, and discovering the delectations of fresh fruits and vegetables.

But cumulatively speaking — by a conservative estimate — America is still *600 million tons overweight.*

And it's not as if we hadn't been *trying.*

"I'm only thirty-eight years old," confides a Cambridge Group Counselor, "and I can tell you that I've already lost 2,156 pounds. And put them all back. And added 17 for good measure. Cambridge, you'd better believe me, was the turnaround in this Loser's Syndrome."

We are such a success-oriented society. So why do we fail — and fail and fail — at something so seemingly simple as taking unwanted, unhealthy, repulsive pounds off our bodies?

We fail because we are misled, again and again, about how best to achieve this desideratum.

Conservative medical opinion would have us believe that any diet that is not reasonably elevated in caloric content is unwise. Conservative medical opinion is reluctant to embrace anything new even after its efficacy has been proved.

Diets, however well-balanced, of 1,000 calories or more are usually self-defeating. After initial weight losses, it is just too tough for most people to stay on them. The increments in weight loss diminish, and there's the feeling, "Why am I giving up so much with so little to show for it?"

At least most doctors subscribe to the concept of the "well-balanced diet."

That is more than can be said for the fad diets that come along to us, each with its fleeting moment in the sun.

One year we are being told we can drink ourselves to stupefaction if we will just remember on the royal road to drunkenness not to eat a baked potato or an apple.

The next year we can have all the lobsters and filet mignons we can ingest. But not much else.

Then it's all the grapefruits we can eat. But that's it.

Or, "If it's Tuesday, I can have six leaves of lettuce and two medallions of veal."

Or, "Any day of the week I may eat unlimited quantities of mangoes, papayas, kiwis, and pomegranates." (Where under the Northern Lights on a glacial winter day do you find fresh-picked papayas in Fargo, North Dakota?)

Or it's those liquid proteins that are minus *complete* protein, and minus almost everything else, that have led too many people almost literally to death's door—if not beyond.

What is wrong, then?

Why are so many of us eternal diet-drifters who never manage to keep off our excess freight?

Because none of these diets works.

Or they work only momentarily.

The reason they do not work is that they are all askew. To put it bluntly, they are wacky. Because they are wacky, they leave the body out of whack. The body is left hungering, hurting for vital nourishment that is missing.

Now at last, out of the laboratories of one of the most prestigious universities in the world, comes this diet that contains every last one of the 50-plus known nutrients the body needs to keep humming along in tiptop shape.

The Cambridge Diet really feeds you. And it does so with such an economy of calories that you will enjoy virtually the results of total fasting while being supremely well-fed.

Thin is in: Fat is out, ugly, and dangerous.

These facts are among the eternal verities.

Fashion is fragile and evanescent; what is chic today is old hat tomorrow.

But in this instance, fashion and chic happen to coalesce with what is right and good for *everybody.*

And this is for keeps.

Never again will being overweight—obesity—be in vogue. Never again will gourmandizing be synonymous with opulence and splendor. Never again will we envy a King Henry VIII or Diamond Jim Brady or King Farouk or William Howard Taft because they have the means to indulge their ravenous appetites.

We are too smart now, too well-informed. We at least know what is best for us.

But knowing what is best for us and transmitting it into decisions at the supermarket and the dinner table can be two different things.

Now we have a diet that makes those decisions so baby-simple.

We have a diet that is quick, versatile, delectable, and gratifying, that produces victories almost instantaneously.

In the Cambridge Diet you will have a good friend for life. You will get rid or those unsightly, life-endangering pounds — and be rid of them forever.

As a lifetime friend Cambridge will be the custodian not only of your weight maintenance but your superlative nutritional well-being.

4

WHAT IS THE CAMBRIDGE DIET?

"Magic in a can!"
    "Almost too good to be true!"
    "The real thing—at last!" .
    "The perfect food—a miracle!"
    "A lifesaver!"
    "THE SOURCE!"
    This praise, comes spontaneously from Cambridge patrons. Particularly those patrons who have been battling being overweight for years, who have gone from one fad diet to the next only to be left with the frustration of defeat.

    Breakthrough—usually an unearned hyperbole—is truly the word for the Cambridge Diet. Is there a more accurate word to describe a diet that brings weight losses almost as rapidly as total fasting or gastroplasty (stapling the stomach) while being nutritionally complete and balanced?

    The Cambridge Diet contains a mere 330 calories a day.

It is a powder scooped from a can and blended with water for three 110-calorie meals.

It is a formula containing protein, carbohydrate, fat, and fiber—in proper proportion to one another—as well as the 33 other nutrients essential to the optimum functioning of the body.

Although consumed in liquid form, the Cambridge Diet is unrelated to those notorious liquid protein diets of yesteryear. *Those* diets consisted of low-grade protein and little else.

The Food and Drug Administration, predictably, has expressed its wariness about this breakthrough; as have some bariatricians (doctors who specialize in weight loss) and nutritionists. In general, the orthodox medical bureaucracy can be expected to look askance at anything innovative that has not been tested for 50 years with three million subjects ranging from rats and mice up through the animal kingdom to *homo sapiens*.

Nobody's health has been put in jeopardy by the Cambridge Diet. Anyone who so alleges is mistaken. Or is someone who should not be on any reducing diet. Or is not telling all. Nobody can be on a very low-calorie diet by day, for example, and then resort to the self-abuse of alcohol or drugs by night without expecting that the system will be thrown into disequilibrium.

The Cambridge Diet is *safe when used as directed*. How could it be otherwise when it supplies the body with everything the body is known to need to keep supremely fortified and supercharged?

The Cambridge Diet comes in ten delectable varieties. These include strawberry, vanilla, eggnog, banana, and chocolate flavors for mixing as a beverage, a double Dutch chocolate dessert that has the consistency of a pudding, and beef, chicken and tomato soups. There is also an herbal salad dressing.

The Cambridge Plan International has been granted worldwide patents; anything else purporting to be "just like Cambridge" is an imposter.

A container of the Cambridge Diet sells for less than one dollar per meal. That's a week's supply of food for one person—three balanced meals daily—at about the cost of one hamburger and a mug of beer at "21."

The Cambridge Diet is not sold in retail outlets.

Sole distribution is through Independent Cambridge Counselors. The Cambridge Diet passes from one hand to another hand, and the hand that passes it is a helping hand.

There may be a Counselor as near as your apartment house or up on the next block. In any event a Counselor is no further away than a toll-free telephone call. Those numbers are: (within California) (800) 682-9261; (outside California) (800) 538-9560.

The Cambridge Diet is made available through The Cambridge Plan International, whose World Headquarters are located on Garden Road, Monterey, California, 93940.

5

GENESIS

In the beginning there was Alan N. Howard, Ph.D., F.R.I.C. (Fellow, Royal Institute of Chemistry).

Dr. Howard is an internationally recognized authority on obesity and cardiovascular diseases. He has headed the Lipid Laboratory of the Department of Medicine of Cambridge University since 1969 and has been with the university for 33 years.

Dr. Howard freely admits that his search for the perfect quick weight-loss diet was inspired in part by enlightened self-interest. Like many people in their late twenties, he was beginning to put on unwanted pounds. Most existing diets, in his opinion, did not really work.

"When people go on 1,000- and 1,500-calorie diets, they lose weight for a short time and then the weight-loss can be painfully slow," he observed. "So I felt that something more effective was needed."

At the time Dr. Howard began looking for some better method of dieting, people with real obesity problems were being put into hospitals — and being put on total fasting regimens. No calories at all. Just water.

There is no question these patients lost lots of weight. But it was at the expense of deteriorating muscle and organ tissue that resulted from the nutritional deficiencies. Somehow, thought Dr. Howard, there must be a happy balance that could be struck between the conventional 1,000- or 1,500-calorie diets of dubious success and the complete deprivation of all food.

The clinical research that led to the development of the Cambridge Diet began in the early 1970s with five severely obese individuals who volunteered to spend a full year in West Middlesex Hospital in London. A primary associate of Dr. Howard in his work on the diet was Ian McLean Baird, M.D., Consulting Physician of West Middlesex and a Fellow of the Royal College of Physicians in London.

Subsequently, some 500 men and women participated in clinical tests under direct medical supervision — both in hospitals and as outpatients — in the United Kingdom and in Holland, Italy, Ireland, and Denmark. All studies corroborated the safety and efficacy of this very low calorie diet. One success followed another.

Early on, Dr. Howard and fellow researchers had two gratifying surprises.

First, contrary to their expectations, they *could* get patients to diet outside a hospital. (The sight of food, of watching other people eat, did not throw their subjects off course and undo all the good work that had begun.) This suggested that they were on to something applicable to millions of people and not just to a relative handful who could be kept under hospital supervision.

Second, there was no need for appetite suppressants. A blind study conducted over a period of eight weeks revealed that a placebo group had fared just as well in continuing to lose weight on the Cambridge Diet as a group taking an additional antiappetite medication. Better, in fact, since the appetite suppressants caused such unpleasant side effects — insomnia, unslakable thirsts — that some of the patients had to stop using them.

The Cambridge Diet in its own right is an appetite suppressant, scientists and doctors concluded. "By having all the nutrients," as Dr. Howard points out, "your body doesn't have any nutritional hunger. It not only reduces the caloric intake, but the ratio of the macronutrients is designed to reduce hunger."

What does the body really need to be completely nourished? In what proportion to one another does it require these vital components? What was the least number of calories that could keep the body properly fed while maximizing weight loss?

These were the big questions that had to be resolved.

It took about two years to complete this research. The intake of protein and carbohydrate had to be revised, and people had to be observed over extended periods of time.

The breakthrough discovery to what Dr. Howard considers a perfect reducing diet presumed finding the minimum amount of protein needed in a very low calorie diet — and the protein-carbohydrate relationship for maintaining nitrogen balance. Nitrogen balance is important because if the body excretes more nitrogen than it is consuming, then lean tissue, rather than fatty tissue, is being broken down to provide calories for energy.

Dr. Howard and his research team made the amazing discovery that 30 grams of protein were "absolutely adequate" for people on a low calorie diet, notwithstanding the general perception that 60 to 70 grams are necessary. "Most overweight people consume more protein than they need," Dr. Howard says.

Further, these researchers discovered that by adding carbohydrate to the diet, the protein needs could be reduced even further. With 30 to 45 grams of carbohydrate, the amount of protein dropped to 15 grams: a daily diet with as few as 180 to 240 calories was feasible!

At the outset, mixtures of purified amino acids were used as the protein source. Then there was a switch to egg protein before the final decision to go with casein and soy proteins, which contain all the essential amino acids. The protein in what became the Cambridge Diet is perfect and complete.

Raising the level of carbohydrate had other beneficial effects. It lowered the blood ketone level, minimizing some of the initial unpleasant effects common to low-calorie diets, such as irritability, diarrhea, and bad breath. The higher level of carbohydrate also helped the body retain electrolytes, potassium, and sodium.

The ideal weight-loss diet then, the scientists concluded, was one that contained slightly more carbohydrate (44 grams) than protein (33 grams). This unique balancing of carbohydrate and protein — as well as fiber, fat, all the U.S. RDA of vitamins and minerals, and all the electrolytes and trace elements specified by the National Academy of Sciences — formed the basis for the patents that have been granted the Cambridge Diet.

The Cambridge Diet was eight and one-half years in the formulating and testing.

It evolved through various stages.

First came the conscientious work and observation in hospitals. Then clinical testing was expanded to include outpatients. During the clinical testing, nine European universities besides Cambridge participated — including the Universities of Rotterdam, Copenhagen, Naples, Gothenburg, and Dublin. Ultimately the formula was modified to 330 calories to lend a margin of safety in protein and carbohydrate to accommodate metabolic differences among individuals.

"It took four to five years to actually work out the formula and to find it was the formula we were looking for," Dr. Howard recalls. "Then it took another two to three years to get the flavors right, seeing that it could be turned into a food that large numbers of people could use and find agreeable."

This is the formula — with its ten flavors — that became the Cambridge Diet.

The results of the exhaustive research that was conducted in England and on the Continent prior to the introduction of the Cambridge Diet in the United States have been published in international professional journals and were discussed at the Third International Congress on Obesity, which was held on the island of Ischia, Italy, in 1980. (See the bibliography.)

The Feather family of California had long been interested in health and self-improvement. They had been successful operators of a chain of slenderizing salons and were now turning their attention to the exploration of nutrition. Wasn't there some better way for millions of people to come to grips with their weight problems than by yo-yoing along from one fad diet to the next, each enjoying its brief season of celebrity, each soon abandoned?

In the spring of 1979, 30,000 feet above the Atlantic Ocean enroute to England, Mr. Jack Feather read an article in the *International Journal of Obesity* on Dr. Howard's dietary breakthrough. He phoned his wife from London saying, "I think I've found what we have been looking for. You'd better come over and we'll meet with Dr. Howard." That meeting resulted in the inception of The Cambridge Plan International in March 1980, with Mrs. Eileen Feather as founder and Mr. Vaughn Feather as president.

6

WEIGH WAY LESS—SWIFTLY!

Everybody loses weight on the Cambridge Diet. It is a biochemical fact that anyone on a 330-calorie-a-day diet loses weight.

It is impossible *not* to lose weight on the Cambridge Diet.

Everybody loses—and wins.

How much weight will you lose? And how fast?

A lot—and very fast.

"We have had one patient who lost nineteen pounds in three days," declares Dr. Robert Birch, who is a staff physician at Summit County Hospital in Coalville, Utah. "This is not all fat loss, of course, but also consists of some body fluids."

How much you lose, and at what tempo, depends on several variables.

Your basic metabolism is a factor. Some people burn up calories, and stored fat, at a faster rate than others.

Gender is a consideration. Overweight men, being generally bigger-framed, tend to drop fat more quickly than overweight women.

If there is a stupendous amount of weight to be shed, it will probably disappear at a brisker clip than if there are a relatively few pounds to go.

But everyone on the Cambridge Diet emerges trimmer, a winner.

Fat is lost every single day when the Cambridge Diet is consumed as the sole source of nutrition.

Routinely men and women testify to having dropped seven and ten and 15 pounds in a week. And 20 or 30 or 40 or more pounds in four short weeks.

But let's let some members of the Cambridge Family speak for themselves.

"I lost 75 pounds in only three and a half months," Bill Gray of Lakewood, Colorado reveals, "but the real accomplishment is that I've kept those pounds off for over two years. I love to eat, which is another reason I love the Cambridge Diet. It lets you enjoy the foods you want, yet maintain your target weight. Now that's the best of both worlds."

Thirty-four-year-old Toni Gossett of Scottsdale, Arizona, confesses that she had been battling with a weight problem for 15 years, especially with heavy thighs. "Then I discovered the Cambridge Diet," she says. "I lost 21 pounds (and inches off my thighs) in only four and a half weeks. That was more than a year ago. I've kept those pounds and inches off and now wear a size four. Today I use the Cambridge Diet for its nutritional value and wouldn't be without it."

Here's Lorrie Otto, 43, of Tigard, Oregon: "I've always been chunky — all my adult life. I was never really fat but not thin. But then I lost 25 pounds on the Cambridge Diet, and I couldn't believe how good I felt, so I lost another five and then another and another. Now I'm 130 pounds, and I've kept off those 40 pounds for more than one year."

"Thanks to the Cambridge Diet," declaims 30-year-old Connie Breedlove of Ventura, California, "I reached my original goal and lost 38 pounds in two months — then continued gradually to a total of forty-four pounds. I have a low metabolism problem. I was wearing size 18 and now wear size eight. I feel so much better. My doctor says I'm healthier than I've ever been."

"I was fat, 40 and a failure," admits Bill Engemann, formerly of the popular singing group, the Lettermen. "Then I went on the Cambridge Diet, and at 41 I was fit and fantastic — and 136 pounds lighter!"

So many of these stories would be heartbreaking but for their happy endings.

On September 12, 1981, Robert Hefflin, a school teacher from Yamhill, Oregon, at six feet eight inches weighed 504 pounds, had high blood pressure (225/165), a rapid pulse (92 beats a minute, resting), a 60-plus waistline, constant headaches, and was always tired. "I felt so bad all the time", recalls Bob, "about ready to die, and my doctor had just about given up on me. I was depressed, irritable and angry, and impossible to live with."

That also happened to be the day that somebody put three cans of chocolate Cambridge into his hands. He lost 300 pounds in about a year! His blood pressure came down to 130/70 and his resting pulse is 58. His waist is a trim 38 inches. His headaches are gone and his disposition is serene.

Bob is not the only Cambridge success in his family. His wife lost 50 pounds, his brother 35 pounds, his daughter 40 pounds, his son 30 pounds. at age 68, his mother lost 52 pounds and has just bought her first pair of designer jeans.

Tom Monroy, an erstwhile advertising agency executive and now one of New York City's most dynamic Group Counselors, is another case in point. Between the spring and the autumn of 1981 he diminished from 312 to 178 pounds!

"That May morning I was going to a meeting and as I stepped out of the cab, my pants split from the inseam to the knees", as Tom remembers it. "My haberdasher told me he could give me another size 48 but that would split too, and if he gave me a 50 it would be too big around the ankles. I came home, took off my clothing and stood in front of a mirror and literally cried. I remember asking myself how I had allowed this to happen to me. I believe that everybody has a responsibility to show up for life and to be in the best physical and mental condition. That night, providentially, a dear friend of mine came to the door bearing three cans of Cambridge. This was the beginning of a new life for me. The big clothes will never be back again, and I have the Cambridge Diet to thank for that."

The five members of the Darrel Miller family — Darrel and his wife Gladys of Ft. Pierce, Florida, daughter Mary Miller Hazellief of Longwood, Florida, daughter Carla of Peoria Heights, Illinois, and son Jeff of Summerville, South Carolina — lost, in the aggregate, an astounding 421 pounds on the Cambridge Diet.

"I'm a registered nurse and night supervisor at a large Medical Center hospital", Gladys Miller tells us. "On January second, 1982, I weighed 255 pounds. At Christmastime we had had a family picture taken; and, even though I'm only 58, I honestly felt it would be the last one because I didn't think I'd live much longer.

"January second is when I started the Cambridge Diet. I lost 39 pounds in 30 days. I had never known such exhilaration. By the end of October, I had lost 105 pounds. My energy level is 100 percent over what is was last January."

Her 62-year-old husband lost 60 pounds and his waistline shriveled from 41 inches to 33 inches. Gladys says that on the diet the aches and pains he had had for years — unsuccessfully diagnosed by doctors — disappeared, and he's gone from being a grouch to someone who's a joy to be around. Daughter Mary's marriage was falling apart because she was having problems and had eaten herself up to 257 pounds; the diet changed all that, and now she and her husband are reconciled. Daugher Carla, an X-ray technician and supervisor in a hospital, lost 100 pounds and has discovered the marvels of dancing and stylish clothing. Navy son Jeff got rid of 30 pounds — and his developing pot. At Christmas 1982 the Miller family got together, had their pictures taken again, and rejoiced at that sizeable fraction of the family that had vanished.

Donna and Clark Ransome of Walnut Creek, California, sponsored and televised a fashion show in the autumn of 1982. The "models" were all men and women who had been on the Cambridge Diet.

There they were, all these gorgeous men and women, in their Pierre Cardins and Bill Blasses and Calvin Kleins and After Sixes, etc. One by one they promenaded across the stage to show off their dazzling new figures. Each in turn stepped to the microphone to relate a personal Cambridge experience:

"I lost 46 pounds in less than two months."

"Cambridge is the eighth wonder of the world."

"Before Cambridge came into my life, I think it had been about 15 years since I had seen my feet."

"I used to go into the back door of clothing stores — I was so ashamed. No more!"

"I've gone from introvert to extrovert. All because I'm no longer disgusted by the way I look."

"Would you believe — I was once a monstrous 34!"

(Cheers, applause and a catcall, "But, baby, look at you now!")

Fashion show or no fashion show the spontaneous expressions of gratitude and affection for Cambridge keep on erupting.

Actress Virginia Pulos: "I had tried Weight Watchers, Scarsdale, Atkins, and lots of other diets, and failed miserably on all of them in one way or another. Here (Cambridge) was one diet that didn't demand that I eat foods I didn't like or, when I was starving, to have to cook....I lost eight pounds in three days and in nine days went from a size 14 to a size ten. I lost 25 pounds all together and went to size six."

Mary Adams, Cumming, Georgia: "Appearance is important to me because as the vice president of general sales of a discount firm, I'm constantly involved in making business contacts and dealing with the public, so I want to look my best....In four weeks on the Cambridge Diet I lost 26 pounds, down from 145 to 119, and went from a zipper-breaking 12 to a stylish six. The Cambridge Diet has not only changed my life, but I really feel it gave me life."

Louisa W. Greaves, Salt Lake City: "Four months after my son was born, I was still 30 pounds overweight. I'm only 24, but I was embarrassed about my appearance and how awful clothes looked on me. I tried to lose weight in so many ways—modified behavior class, the kind of diet they gave to diabetics, just eating one salad a day and drinking diet drinks. They all were such a hassle. I'd start on one, stay on it a couple of days, then hate it and quit. The Cambridge Diet is the first nutritional diet I'd ever used. I lost eight pounds in the first three days and a total of 32 pounds and went from a size 15 to a size seven. My husband is really excited about the way I look."

Melanee Wood, of Ft. Pierce, Florida: "On August first, 1981, I weighed 422 pounds on the hospital laundry scales, and my doctor told me I was definitely going to die if I didn't do something about my weight. I was 20 years old and too young to die.

"I slept on two mattresses on the floor because no bed would hold me. I was propped up on five pillows, in a near sitting position so I could breathe, and I had to hold my chest down or the fat would roll over my mouth and nose and I would suffocate. When I sat in a chair, my stomach literally went over my knees....Every day I would go to McDonald's and order two quarter-pounders with cheese, two filet sandwiches, two fries, and two cokes. Then I'd drive around the corner to Kentucky Fried Chicken and order double servings of five-piece boxes, with double fries and two more cokes. If I was really hungry, I'd go on to Burger King and double up a third time....My mother had lost 130 pounds on the Cambridge Diet, and she begged me to try it and get the pressure off my heart. So I started on the Cambridge Diet, and in six months I'd lost 100 pounds. Now, in 18 months, I've lost 251 pounds, weigh 171, and I'm still losing."

Kenneth W. Winright, of Temple Terrace, Florida: "I never thought

I'd learn how to lose weight from my veterinarian, but at 251 pounds I guess I *was* becoming as big as a horse. He told me about the Cambridge Diet, and I lost 80 pounds in only 120 days."

Linda Stern Greenberg of Annapolis, Maryland: "I am a tiny (just five feet) woman who works with miniature horses as a hobby, but I used to weigh over 170 pounds. For years I had been trying every diet that came down the pike. While I was on a 'banana diet' a friend told me about Cambridge, and I said, 'Oh, no, not *another* fad diet', but I was sick of bananas and decided I had nothing to lose. But I did. I lost 60 pounds on the Cambridge Diet and went from wearing some size 22 pants to wearing a sleek size two, and now I show off my figure everywhere I go. My mother at age 74 now looks 50 years old thanks to Cambridge and the 55 pounds she has lost."

Karen S. Thomas of Columbus, Ohio: "After my daughter was born last March, I just couldn't lost those 20 pounds. The Cambridge Diet helped me lose 18 pounds in less than four weeks and made me much more aware of the importance of good nutrition.

Sandy Sanders, Ashland, Kentucky: "I lost 25 pounds in two weeks on the Cambridge Diet—and I couldn't believe my eyes. I used to look like the Goodyear blimp and bought clothes to cover my bulging middle and to hide my double chin. My husband told me point blank he didn't want a fat wife—and believe you me, now that I know about the Cambridge Diet, he'll never have one."

S. Byron Wareham, D.D.S., Anderson, California: "I lost 25 pounds quickly and easily on the Cambridge Diet, my waist went from 38 inches to 34 inches, and my blood pressure dropped from 160/100 to 120/78, which truly pleased and impressed my physician. I feel great, and I'm committed to the Cambridge Plan for the rest of my life."

Charles Chatham, Winston-Salem, North Carolina: "I lost 14 pounds in five days on the Cambridge Diet—and then I went on vacation with Cambridge in my suitcase, and I continued to have it three times a day while enjoying all the fresh seafood I could eat. I didn't gain any weight. When I got home, I lost another 11 pounds in one week. The change in my appearance and attitude became apparent to everybody, and the reaction of my family and friends to the 'new me' has been terrific. I'm enjoying life and everything else so much more."

Irene Smith, of Dallas: "I am 60 years old and have had a weight problem for years. I was on a doctor's weight program for four years and lost the same 50 pounds four times. That was so frustrating. I was a secretary, and every time I lost the weight, I would go back to my old routine of large lunches and sitting all day and gain the weight right back. Finally, my doctor, who had heard of the Cambridge Diet from another doctor who was taking the diet himself, recommended I go on the Plan and said he would monitor me. He also asked me to keep a diary of my experience. I started losing weight right away, and I have now lost 70 pounds. My doctor still can't believe it. No more depression, no more feelings of uselessness, just healthy, happy, and ready to live to be 100!"

Says Doreen Betts of Elk Grove, California: "We're a Cambridge Diet family. I lost 30 pounds, and my husband lost 50. I lost weight all over, but what really excited me was that most of it came off my hips and thighs, where I carried most of my extra pounds.

"But I can't say enough about how the Cambridge Diet helped my ten-year-old daughter. She has always had a tendency to be a somewhat hyperactive child. Now that she's been having the Cambridge Diet three times a day as a nutritional supplement, I've noticed a big difference in her. She's calmed down tremendously."

Jennifer Shober, of Sacramento: "When he hears the blender going, our three-year-old son will come running into the kitchen and ask for some Cambridge. It doesn't matter if it's Cambridge with water, Cambridge with milk, or Cambridge pudding. He just loves it. We divide one scoopful three ways. We feel we're not only giving him something that he enjoys but also something that's nutritious and good for him, too."

Linda McLaughlin of Chicago had had a weight problem for about nine years. She had been following the example of her mother and trying every new diet—even fasting, diet pills, and spending $600.00 at a diet clinic. Everything failed and she was afraid she was "doomed to being fat forever!" Then while visiting a friend in Phoenix one week-end she discovered Cambridge.

"I lost 21 pounds in less than a month on sole source," Linda reports, "then I went on maintenance for about a week, then lost 19 more pounds on sole source. I lost five inches in my bustline, five inches in my waistline, six inches from my hips, and eight inches totally from my thighs which have always been the biggest problem for me. I went from a size 13 or 15 dress to a size 7. I've never felt better!"

Richard S. Frezza, Memphis, Tennessee, recalls: "When I went on the Cambridge Diet I weighed 256 pounds. I lost 86 pounds so fast that physicians at the hospital where I was employed as a nurse anesthetist were concerned about how rapidly I was losing weight and asked if they might

23

run some tests. Periodically they ran a SMAC (Simultaneous Multiple Analyzer-C) and were so impressed with the improvement that soon many of them and/or their families were also drinking the Cambridge formula.

"More important than the weight loss is the change in my health. Three years ago I had a cardiac catherization and was told I was a prime candidate for the 'pump' (coronary care) room. I felt awful, tense, and upset most of the time, had hypertension and tachycardia; my cholesterol and triglyceride levels were off the page. Now I feel great, *everything* is normal, and my triglyceride level shows that I am a zero risk factor.

"I am personally committed to the Cambridge Plan, not only for dieting but for lifetime nutrition."

And on and on and on into the blue horizon.

The affidavits to lost weight and found lives are beyond counting.

We are all potential models in the fashion show of the Ransomes or any other fashion show someone may be sponsoring.

We can all lose pounds and pounds and pounds — and prontissimo — on the Cambridge Diet.

("When I was one-and-twenty I heard a wise man say," wrote the poet A.E. Housman in *A Shropshire Lad,* "give crowns and *pounds* (italics ours) and guineas, but not your heart away.")

The name of the most democratic, all-inclusive, all-benefits-shared club in the world?

The Cambridge Family.

7

THE INDISPENSABLE COUNSELOR

The Cambridge Counselor is a person of *invaluable* importance to any patron on the Cambridge Diet.

The Counselor is a person *who has been there.*

The Counselor is a new friend in your life.

He/she cares about you.

Think of the Counselor as a surrogate big brother/big sister.

No one needs to be a medical doctor or a psychotherapist or a dietician to be a Counselor.

The essence of effective counseling is having had a personal, unique experience with the Cambridge Diet—and being "high" on it from that experience.

Counselors—and now there are upwards of 200,000 of them—cut across all socio-economic-professional cleavages. Many of them just happen to be doctors and psychotherapists and dieticians. But among the others are schoolteachers, accountants, dentists, salesmen, homemakers, actors, domestics, social workers, mailmen, nurses, athletes, librarians, corporate executives, carpenters, bus drivers, veterinarians, editors and publishers, film makers, agents, writers, clerks, secretaries, farmers, and merchants.

The Cambridge Family of Counselors is a microcosm of American society at large.

"Caring and sharing" is virtually inscribed on the cornerstone of Cambridge Plan International.

Dieting undertaken on one's own can be a lonely, fearful experience. But Cambridge is so different.

The Cambridge Counselor substantively leads the patron by the hand through the whole weight-loss program — and beyond.

There is always someone there for you as the patron. There is someone who is interested in your progress, who can answer questions, dispel doubts, and express encouragement and congratulations.

The Counselor, or course, keeps the patron supplied with the Cambridge Diet.

But that is only the beginning of the Counselor's responsibility.

The Counselor shares his/her own exhilarating success on the Cambridge Diet.

The Counselor holds regular meetings at which patrons share *their* experiences, and these characteristically become joyous, mutually supportive occasions.

In addition to the support role, the conscientious Counselor can be a resource of nutritional information. "Your body needs Vitamin B6 for cholesterol management." "We all need selenium to reinforce cell membranes and promote growth and fertility." (And we need some 50 other nutrients, and they are all here — macronutrients and micronutrients in perfect configuration — in the Cambridge Diet.)

In his Waterside Plaza apartment, 33 floors above the East River, Manhattan Group Counselor Ronald Dobrin, who is also a novelist and a film maker, had this telephone conversation one January afternoon with a patron:

"How many pounds did you lose yesterday? Two? Excellent! I wish my arms were long enough to reach out and give you a big hug. No headaches? Good!

"What dress size are you now? 14? And you want to get to eight? If you have a little free time in the next day or two, why don't you go up to Bloomingdale's or Saks and look at dresses in the size you're going to wear. Even try one on to see how close you are to fitting into it. You're going to be wearing that size eight so fast you won't believe it!

"Here's another thing. When you start your period, don't get discouraged by what the scales tell you. The body retains fluid at that time, and it may seem that you are not making progress. But you are. You'll be losing fat all that time, and afterwards when you weigh yourself you'll be in for a beautiful surprise."

After hanging up the phone, Ron reflected, "You know, I would never have dreamed I could be this personal with someone I've just met. But this is different. You really feel so close to people and whatever they may be experiencing. This is just something totally different. We all know how most of the business world operates. But with Cambridge it's something else. You do something for somebody and it comes back a hundredfold."

Counselor Jacqui Bishop of White Plains, New York, a psychotherapist, says, "I call a new patron the first day if at all possible, and I stay with that patron on a daily basis until he's passed through the transition period. That's the period during which he's shifting his fuel economy: instead of taking the bulk of his calories from outside his body, he's taking them from his own fat stores. Most people, by the second or third time I call, say, 'Hey, I'm really doing great! I have more energy than I've had in years. I'd like my mom (dad, friend, boss) to go on it. I'll bring them Wednesday night to the meeting. Okay?'

"Another thing: I avoid talking about *losing* weight, because whatever's lost we tend to try to find again. Instead I talk about *getting rid of* pounds and inches."

No one sums up the function of the Counselor better than Suzanne Wade (who lost 125 pounds and kept them off) of Livermore, California, when she says, "My personal experience is a vital part of my role as a Cambridge Counselor. As a Cambridge Counselor, I have seen many patrons stay on the program as a direct result of the personal support and understanding which they receive from *peers* who have *been there* and who are committed to helping others succeed. Dieting can be very frustrating, but a helping hand along the way can make the difference between success and failure.

"I believe that one of the greatest strengths that the Cambridge Diet offers is the total removal of conventional food while using the Cambridge Diet as the sole source of nutrition. In addition, the Cambridge Diet program permits *real behavior modification* during the 'Add-a-Meal' transition to lifetime balanced nutrition. This basic *change in eating habits* and philosophy is essential if the patron is to maintain his weight loss."

Caroline Bliss-Isberg, a 40 pounds lighter Cambridge Counselor—

also from California — with a Ph.D. in special education, echoes these sentiments:

"My life has always been geared toward ways of helping others. I have a masters in speech pathology from Stanford University and founded what turned out to be the largest special education unit in the country: Idylwild Center for Communicative Disorders in Santa Clara County. After I finished my doctorate, I was working at the University of California in Berkeley and had gained about 40 pounds. I looked and felt terrible, and finally my mother brought me some Cambridge Diet. She told me she had been taking it for a year, and though I had been too busy to notice, she had lost 20 pounds and had more energy than I had! I argued with her for about half an hour, being an intellectual snob who simply was *not* going to use a fad diet, before I gave in and said I would try it for three days. On the fourth day I called her to ask what was in it; I felt fantastic and had lost seven pounds already.

"I started ordering Cambridge regularly, and as my students at Cal watched me go from a size 14 to a size eight in only one month, they started asking me about it and how to get it. Also, my husband Cliff had taken a month's trip to Japan, and when I saw his plane off I was a dumpy 14. When I picked him up again, I was wearing size eight designer jeans, and he was just blown away! My mother decided to become a Cambridge Counselor, and when I realized that I was actually spending a great deal of time counseling other people on the diet anyway, and I was doing something I really enjoyed, I decided to become a Counselor, too.

"To be a Counselor, you don't need to be an expert or professional person, but you do need to care deeply about the welfare of the people you are counseling and make every effort to help other people experience the same benefits of good nutrition that you have experienced. Dieting is very personal, and positive personal contact with someone who wants to help you succeed can form a very strong bond between Counselor and patron."

The Cambridge Counselor is someone who is required to have been on the diet for a minimum of two weeks for the motivations of either weight reduction or improved nutrition.

The Cambridge Counselor is the friend to someone in need who is also that friend in deed.

The Counselor is someone who *knows,* who in effect says to the Cambridge "baby," "We're all in this together. Welcome to the family."

Look for this Logo of Independent Cambridge Counselors

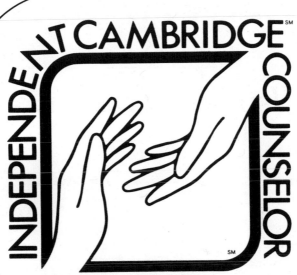

- **LIFETIME NUTRITION**
- **UNPARALLELED WEIGHT LOSS**
- **PERSONALIZED COUNSELING**

Servicemark of Cambridge Plan International
© Copyright Cambridge Plan International 1983 • All rights reserved

550103

8

WELL MET IN CAMBRIDGE

The Cambridge meetings!

All over America people are coming to the meetings. Regularly. In the hundreds of thousands.

People come to Cambridge meetings in multiples of 8, 16, 124 — or more.

The atmosphere is chummy, clubby.

If most of the patrons are relatively new to Cambridge, the Counselor or a visiting doctor may offer a nutritional briefing. "Electrolytes serve extremely important functions in the body. Among the electrolytes are sodium, potassium, calcium, and chloride, and they are all found in balanced quantities in the Cambridge Diet."

"What is ketosis?" someone may ask.

"Incomplete breakdown of fat occurs when the carbohydrate supply is limited and leads to the formation of ketones. When these substances are present in the urine we are said to be in a state of ketosis. Severe ketosis can bring on headaches, dizziness, aggressiveness and insomnia. With the

Cambridge Diet most people have a small amount of ketosis, leading in some cases to a feeling of mild euphoria, a state of well-being, which is advantageous to people on a weight loss diet."

From around the living room — or the auditorium, or the banquet hall or the executive suite — come the testimonials.

"My name is____and I've been on the Cambridge Diet eleven days, and I've already lost 16 pounds."

Applause.

"My name is ____and I've lost 19 pounds in less than three weeks on the Cambridge Diet, and I would like everyone to know I've never felt so wonderful in all my life. I couldn't believe I'd ever have so much energy."

Applause.

"Hi, I'm____and I want to tell you I went on the Cambridge Diet for strictly nutritional purposes. But do you want to know something? *Incidentally,* I lost 106 pounds!"

Laughter *and* applause.

"If I didn't know better, I'd suspect this powder was laced with amphetamines — I feel so *up* all the time!"

Applause and chuckles of recognition.

Confidences and confessionals are exchanged.

"I feel so virtuous. Today is my birthday, and my best friend popped up on my doorstep with a big chocolate cake. I thanked her profusely and didn't touch a morsel of it. Two minutes in the mouth. An hour or so working its way through the alimentary canal. *Forever* on the hips."

"I don't know when anything has ever so united my whole family. We're *all* on Cambridge. Including Sir Winston, our overweight English bulldog."

"My three-year-old son is hooked on the strawberry. Okay, so he's going to be a Cambridge strawberry milk shake freak. As a mother, I can't think of anything better for him to be on."

"Next week I expect to squeeze into a size seven. That's a place, believe me, I haven't been since I was about 16."

"I put about a teaspoon of the salad dressing in either the tomato or the chicken soup, and it gives the soup a nice extra tangy little edge."

"I trot out the crystal and the sterling silver soup toureens. Goodness, this is an *occasion,* dropping all these pounds. Why not put on the dog a little bit while we're doing it? I use my best goblets for the chocolate dessert."

And the beat goes on.

"I cheated today," a remorseful woman confesses. "This is only my second day and I felt so —."

"Excuse me, Samantha," interrupts the Counselor. "So you did. In the beginning we have to be a little patient with ourselves. We are attempting a significant break with the past. We all know what that is. Who of us who have been on diets all our lives can't remember days when we would have gladly turned in our Braque for a beefburger? It is very difficult to go 'cold turkey' with bad, overeating habits. It may take the system a little while to adapt to perfect nutrition. It may be, too, Samantha, that your subconscious was telling you that you must have this or that. So you had whatever it was. Today. And perhaps tomorrow you'll feel you don't need any extra food to supplement the totally adequate nutrition you are getting with the three Cambridge meals."

Someone comments, "I have a friend who claimed she had been on the Cambridge Diet for days and hadn't lost any weight. I told her that was impossible."

"You told her right."

"I asked her, just trying to be helpful but not nosey, to keep a log for one day of everything she put into her mouth besides the three Cambridge meals. Well, she did, and it turns out she's been working a lot of overtime at her office down on Wall Street and downing cup after cup of coffee to keep alert. I asked her if she took anything in her coffee, and she told me half-and-half and three teaspoons of sugar!"

"And she would swear she's not eating anything besides the Cambridge meals," responds the Counselor. "What we must all realize is that calories, in whatever disguise, are food. We are, practically speaking, eating even when we consume a seemingly innocuous beverage if that beverage contains any form of sugar or dairy products."

Going down the elevator a patrician, silver-haired lady gurgles, "I know this will date me. But I'm reminded of that old popular song that goes 'If that isn't love it'll have to do until the real thing comes along.'"

The Cambridge meetings.

Brotherhood and sisterhood.

Stroking and soothing.

Caring and sharing.

9

CAUTIONARY NOTE

It is axiomatic that anyone planning to go on any kind of weight-loss program should first consult with his or her doctor. Anyone who is under a physician's care for some chronic condition or is on regular medication is certainly well advised to seek medical permission – and supervision during the diet.

By consulting physicians and having their progress monitored during the course of the diet, Cambridge patrons already under medical care will be assured that while their weight decreases, their general health conditions will be monitored by a knowledgeable professional. Thus, appropriate adjustments can be made in medication and other treatment procedures.

All Cambridge product literature and the product containers carry this counsel:

"Consult your doctor before starting this diet. In particular, individuals who have heart and cardiovascular conditions, stroke, kidney disease, diabetes, gout, hypoglycemia, chronic infections, the very elderly, growing children, adolescents, or anyone under medical care for any other condition should diet only under medical supervision. Your doctor can advise you whether you have any of the above conditions or for any reason you should not be on this or any other diet. Pregnant women and nursing mothers should not be on any weight-loss program.

"The Cambridge Diet formula is designed for use as a sole source of nutrition for periods of not to exceed four consecutive weeks at any time."

10

A DIET BY ANY OTHER NAME IS *NOT* CAMBRIDGE

Another of the ineluctable facts of life is that the ripoff artists, alas, are always among us.

Imitation may be the sincerest form of flattery, but an imitation is just that.

Be it said for the imitators, they at least recognize a great thing when they see it. They have even tried to identify with the academic prestige of Cambridge University by calling themselves things like the Oxford Diet or the University Diet. Next week, the Harvard Diet. Or the Yale Diet.

"Having trouble finding the Cambridge Diet?" placards hail us from the windows of drug stores and health food emporiums. "Try us. We're just as good."

The truth is they are not as good.

Because of The Cambridge Plan International patents, no one can copy the diet exactly. So the would-be copiers must add things or leave out things and that makes it a different diet—and an untested one.

Mr. Jack Feather has a favorite word for the imitators. Epigones. An epigone is an undistinguished and inferior copier of an important original.

Dr. Alan N. Howard worked with a team of medical doctors at Cambridge all those years testing and refining the diet to make it a thing of perfection — a diet that would contain every element essential to sound nutrition and contain these elements in flawless balance. And then deliver that diet with a minimum of calories.

The diet formulations that aspire to plug into the glory of Cambridge are doomed to second-class status.

No other diet has the support network of counselors who are there to insure that every patron turns up a winner.

There is only one Cambridge Diet. Any other diet claiming "sameness" is something else — an unknown quantity.

11

TAKING THE HIGH ROAD
TO CAMBRIDGE

You've heard/read it here, there and everywhere.

"The Cambridge Diet is a miracle worker...dynamite!"

You too want to join the millions who have already been to Cambridge.

You have your doctor's blessing to go on a very low calorie diet.

You want to go on this diet that promises *maximum* nutrition and *minimum* calories.

And one that promises safety and victory.

Some Counselors speak of the three C's associated with Cambridge. Compassion. Contact. Celebration.

You have compassion for yourself obviously because you are about to do something tremendous for yourself. And that compassion will be mutual among you and others who will be sharing in this salubrious new adventure.

There is always contact with others on this diet. The Counselor is just a phone call away and will be monitoring your progress. There are the

Cambridge meetings to go regularly where patrons exchange experiences and revelations and helpful suggestions. ("Before Cambridge took me out of my humdrum existence", declares a Chicago man, "I had no friends and now it seems I've got about a thousand!")

The celebration begins almost immediately and never quits. Because the results are instantaneous and go on and on.

While people with a great deal of weight to lose are advised not to stay on the Cambridge Diet as a sole source of their nutrition for more than 28 days, actually most of us could easily tolerate the diet for more than 28 days. But this restriction provides a margin of safety. (Many's the person who has adapted exceedingly well to total fasts — water only — for 30 or 40 days and longer.)

A fourth Cambridge "C" could stand for commitment.

In the beginning it's best to commit yourself to a time goal — some number of days or weeks you are going at least to try very earnestly to stick with the diet.

Some solicitous Counselors will say to a prospective patron, "I am not going to let you have any product until you first come to a meeting. I want you to be thoroughly convinced you mean to go on this diet and stay the course."

One week seems a logical choice of minimum commitment because each can of the Cambridge Diet contains a week's supply of meals.

In every can there is a scoop. Place a level scoop in eight ounces of water and blend. You may use hot or cold water. You may blend Cambridge with ice, with extracts or spices for extra flavor, with sugar substitutes, with diet drinks or coffee. (See the delicious recipes for Cambridge product meals developed in the Cambridge Kitchens.)

Consume three Cambridge meals each day.

You also must drink a minimum of eight glasses of water every day. This is most important. Humankind has been known to survive prodigious amounts of time without food, but not without water. Water is part of the weight-reducing process; it prevents dehydration because of all the water-heavy foods that are not being eaten, and it flushes out the toxins. While water does not contain calories or vitamins, it does provide minerals, and therefore it must be considered as a nutrient that is vital to life. Also, drinking the water will help stave off any possible sensations of hunger, particularly during the first day or so of the diet.

In addition, you may drink tea, black coffee (no sugar or cream or cream substitutes), mineral water, and diet sodas. But remember that diet sodas and sparkling waters contain sodium and this may cause water retention—as well as being unadvisable for people with elevated blood pressure. Coffee, tea, and some diet sodas, because of the caffeine, are recommended in moderation too; too many stimulants can be unnerving to a body whose systems are coming into a state of grace and tranquility.

Alcohol contains calories and for this and other reasons is emphatically a no-no while on this diet.

May you exercise? Definitely yes. Exercise can only accelerate the reducing process as well as being generally health enhancing. Newly discovered reservoirs of energy will make most people *feel* like exercising. Perhaps the best form of exercise during the dieting period is brisk walking. Use common sense. Listen to your body!

You should weigh yourself each morning before you've had your Cambridge meal or any water or other beverages. Today, another two pounds gone! Every morning, another success.

Also measure yourself regularly. You'll be losing inches along with pounds—and losing them where you most wanted to lose them. Sooner than soon you'll have the figure you always wanted but never dared dream would be yours.

The first day or two can be the hardest. But many, many Cambridge patrons sail straight through from hour one without a twinge of hunger or a second of unpleasantness.

One suggestion, if there is some initial feeling of hunger, is to divide the three Cambridge meals into six minimeals. And another is to drink more water.

Any minor side effects—headaches or dizziness—should be transitory.

Mind-set in this experience, as in all aspects of life, can be the key to success.

Positive thinking about the goals of weight loss, glamorized appearance, and the boost toward improved health and vitality should carry the day through any temporary malaise.

The thing to remember is that the Cambridge Diet is thoroughly nourishing you. Of course, everybody requires more than the 330 calories the diet provides to keep going. For those extra calories you are living off the fat of the body. Or "the blob and bloat," as a Minneapolis businessman phrases it.

No one should take less than the three Cambridge meals a day. But there are instances when people expending huge amounts of energy—laborers and athletes, to take two examples—may want to consume a fourth meal.

Sometimes a plateau of apparent nonprogress may be reached. No change on the scales for a day or two or three. That plateau is misleading. The weight-loss campaign is advancing all the while. The body may be retaining water temporarily, as during menstrual cycles, and this accounts for what seems like discouraging news but isn't.

There is another kind of plateau that sometimes manifests itself in the end stretch. It has been called the Last Ten Pounds Syndrome. Some people will lose pounds and pounds and pounds and come so near to their ideal weight — that goal they have been dreaming of achieving — and then there is a resistance.

Chancellor Group Counselor Sandy Kellen of Phoenix, a member of the U.S. bobsledding team that made it to the finals in the Winter Olympics at Lake Placid, New York, illustrates the point with this case history:

"There was a woman who had lost about a hundred pounds. She maybe had twenty more to lose. But there she stopped. Something was holding her back from going that last mile. It was suggested to her that she hold a wake for that self she had lost, all those pounds. She should even put on mourning clothes. Then when she was done grieving, she could take off the mourning clothes. Then she'd be able to finish the journey. And that's what happened."

That story is typical of the innovativeness with which Cambridge Counselors in their concern for patrons resolve problems and push away stumbling blocks.

The pages of *Our World,* the Cambridge Plan publication, abound with news of 50-Pound Clubs and 100-Pound Clubs (lost pounds) springing up around the country. There are Before and After pictures of people who look to be about one-third the size of their former selves. The message is explicit: if these many people can do it, then this is do-able by anyone with the will to do it.

And now there is the perfect way to do it.

12

DELICIOUS CAMBRIDGE PRODUCT RECIPES

Developed in the Cambridge Kitchens, the eight yummy flavorings in the following recipes contain no sugar, are nonalcoholic, and very low in calories. More flavorings on the way from Cambridge!

Mocha Creme

    1 scoop vanilla Cambridge formula
    ¾ cup cold water
    3 or more ice cubes
    1 teaspoon decaffeinated coffee
    Low-calorie sweetener equal to 1 teaspoon sugar

    (Combine in blender and mix until smooth)

Strawberry Pineapple

    1 scoop strawberry Cambridge formula
    ¾ cup cold water
    3 or more ice cubes
    ¼ teaspoon pineapple flavor
    Low-calorie sweetener equal to 1 teaspoon sugar

(Combine in blender and mix until smooth)

Strawberry Coconut

    1 scoop strawberry Cambridge formula
    ¾ cup cold water
    3 or more ice cubes
    ¼ teaspoon coconut flavor
    ¼ teaspoon vanilla flavor
    Low-calorie sweetener equal to 1 teaspoon sugar

(Combine in blender and mix until smooth)

Banana Walnut

    1 scoop banana Cambridge formula
    ¾ cup cold water
    3 or more ice cubes
    ¼ teaspoon black walnut flavor
    Low-calorie sweetener equal to 1 teaspoon sugar

(Combine in blender and mix until smooth)

Holiday Eggnog

1 scoop eggnog Cambridge formula
1 cup hot or cold water
¼ teaspoon brandy flavor
¼ teaspoon rum flavor
¼ teaspoon vanilla flavor
Low-calorie sweetener equal to 1 teaspoon sugar

(Combine in blender and mix until smooth)

Strawberry Shortcake

1 scoop strawberry Cambridge formula
¾ cup cold water
3 or more ice cubes
¼ teaspoon vanilla flavor
Low-calorie sweetener equal to 1 teaspoon sugar

(Combine in blender and mix until smooth)

Chocolate Ice Cream

½ scoop Cambridge chocolate dessert formula
½ scoop Cambridge chocolate drink formula
2 oz. chilled water
4-6 ice cubes
¼ teaspoon almond flavor
Low-calorie sweetener equal to 1 teaspoon sugar

(Combine in blender until smooth)
Pour well-blended ingredients into ice cream maker and churn until frozen yoghurt consistency or harder; 10–15 minutes.

Tropical Fruit Ice Cream

1 scoop strawberry Cambridge formula
¾ cup cold water
¼ teaspoon coconut flavor
¼ teaspoon pineapple flavor
¼ teaspoon banana flavor
¼ teaspoon rum flavor
Low-calorie sweetener equal to 2 teaspoons sugar

(Combine in blender and mix until smooth)
Pour well-blended ingredients into ice cream maker and churn until frozen yoghurt consistency or harder; 10–15 minutes.

Double Chicken Soup

1 scoop chicken soup Cambridge formula
1 cup *hot* water
⅛ teaspoon poultry seasoning
¼ teaspoon (scant) onion powder
⅛ teaspoon nutmeg
⅛ teaspoon (scant) garlic powder
¼ teaspoon butter flavor

(Combine in blender and mix until smooth)

Souped-Up Tomato Soup

1 scoop tomato soup Cambridge formula
1 cup *hot* water
1 teaspoon lemon juice
½ teaspoon dried basil, crumbled
½ teaspoon dried thyme, crumbled
¼ teaspoon onion powder
¼ teaspoon butter flavor

(Combine in blender until smooth)

Curried Chicken Soup

1 scoop chicken soup Cambridge formula
1 cup *hot* water
½ teaspoon curry powder
½ teaspoon onion powder
½ teaspoon dried parsley
¼ teaspoon butter flavor
Optional: pinch of black pepper

(Combine in blender until smooth)

Pizza Soup

1 scoop tomato soup Cambridge formula
1 cup *hot* water
dash tobasco sauce
⅛ teaspoon onion powder
⅛ teaspoon garlic powder
¼ teaspoon butter flavor
¼ teaspoon Italian herbs
Optional: pinch of black pepper

(Combine in blender until smooth)

Vanilla Almond

1 scoop vanilla Cambridge formula
¾ cup cold water
3 or more ice cubes
¼ teaspoon vanilla flavor
¼ teaspoon almond flavor
Low-calorie sweetener equal to ½ teaspoon sugar

(Combine ingredients in blender and mix until smooth)

Jamoca Almond Fudge

1 scoop chocolate Cambridge formula
¾ cup cold water
3 or more ice cubes
1 teaspoon instant coffee
¼ teaspoon almond flavor
Low-calorie sweetener equal to 1 teaspoon sugar

(Combine in blender and mix until smooth)

Chocolate Banana Split

½ scoop chocolate Cambridge formula
½ scoop banana Cambridge formula
¾ cup cold water
3 or more ice cubes
¼ teaspoon banana flavor
Low-calorie sweetener equal to ½ teaspoon sugar

(Combine in blender and mix until smooth)

Cambridge Cappuccino

1 scoop vanilla Cambridge formula
¾ cup *hot* water
1 teaspoon instant decaffeinated coffee
¼ teaspoon rum flavor
⅛ teaspoon cinnamon flavor
Low-calorie sweetener to equal ½ teaspoon sugar

(Combine in blender and mix until smooth)

Coconut Almond Fudge

1 scoop chocolate Cambridge formula
¾ cup cold water
3 or more ice cubes
¼ teaspoon coconut flavor
¼ teaspoon almond flavor
Low-calorie sweetener to equal ½ teaspoon sugar

(Combine in blender and mix until smooth)

Pineapple Crush

1 scoop vanilla Cambridge formula
¾ cup cold water
3 or more ice cubes
¼ teaspoon pineapple flavor
¼ teaspoon coconut flavor
Low-calorie sweetener to equal ½ teaspoon sugar

(Combine in blender and mix until smooth)

Banana Coconut Freeze

1 scoop banana Cambridge formula
¾ cup cold water
3 or more ice cubes
¼ teaspoon banana flavor
¼ teaspoon coconut flavor
Low-calorie sweetener to equal ½ teaspoon sugar

(Combine in blender and mix until smooth)

13

LOST LABORS, FOUND TIME

There's so much less work and extra leisure for the Cambridge patron.

For the time being, no more pushing shopping carts through supermarket aisles and queueing up at the checkout counter.

No more time-consuming preparation of meals. Or planning of menus. Or washing up in the kitchen.

The Cambridge Diet is the epitome of simplicity. It's so easy. It's so quick to whip up.

Ace Hollywood agent Marty Ingels and his beautiful wife actress Shirley Jones relate this amusing tale:

The Ingels heard about the Cambridge Diet from a ski instructor. Marty decided he would like to drop a fast 25 pounds and his wife kept him company on the Cambridge Diet, dropping a few of her own to become even more beautiful. Prior to their going on the diet they had been having a minor labor dispute with the cook who was importuning for a wage increase. Came the Cambridge Diet with the Ingels having their simple, easy, no-mess

Cambridge breakfasts, lunches, and dinners, and the cook dropped the whole discussion about salary!

(The Ingels, incidentally, went on the "Tattletales" television program hosted by Bert Convy, sipping their Cambridge beverages. According to Marty, in the entertainment business today it's "in to be thin," and a lot of the Hollywood biggies who have been getting a little too big in the wrong places are getting rid of their excess pounds and inches with the Cambridge Diet.)

Cambridge time is a time to use all the gained hours to excellent advantage. There are all those books and movies that have been waiting for those hunks of discretionary leisure that have been so elusive.

It is *not* a time that is best spent watching much television. Commercial TV is hugely supported by manufacturers/processors of food and beverage products we would do well to avoid even when we are not on a diet. This is a time when we should try to keep our minds off eating, and looking at representations of food is no help.

Besides, you will have so much new-found energy that you will want to be more active.

This is a time for long walks—but no browsing at menus posted in restaurant windows.

This is a time to go to museums, to start a new hobby, to catch up with neglected friends.

Being on the Cambridge Diet should be no deterrent to keeping up with one's social life. The nondrinker finds it easy to say, "I'll have tonic water and lime or a Virgin Mary or a Shirley Temple." Nobody can force food on you that you have chosen not to eat. You can, with impunity, take your Cambridge meal to someone else's house when invited there to dinner. Friends are most understanding when we make a commitment to do something to better ourselves.

You can even go out to lunch. Yes. People are doing it anyway in some of Manhattan's plushiest beaneries. They're taking their Cambridge meal to places like the Water Club and the Four Seasons and sipping it with the greatest of ease and enjoyment. (The Perrier they order, of course, may set them back a few bucks.)

14

"FOOD, WONDERFUL FOOD!"

So sang Oliver Twist in the Broadway musical *Oliver.*

Say we all.

No diet — particularly a very low calorie diet — can be endured forever.

No one should stay on the Cambridge Diet as a sole source of nutrition longer than four consecutive weeks.

How does one come off the Cambridge Diet?

Very safely and very sensibly.

The best advice is to stay with the three Cambridge formula meals every day. And add a 400-calorie meal.

The chefs and the dieticians in the Cambridge Kitchens have created luscious, nutritous meals with varying caloric contents. (For a sampling of 400-calorie meals see Cambridge Cuisine.)

Poulet a l'orange, anyone? Or Beef Stroganoff with noodles and lima beans and carrots? Or Frittata with fruit compote? Or Poached Sole Julienne? They all weigh in at a mere 400 calories.

On the three Cambridge meals a day and an additional 400-calorie meal, most people will keep on losing weight.

If there are substantial amounts more of weight to be lost, then after a week of this regimen of three Cambridge meals *plus* a 400-calorie meal, it is time to resume the Cambridge as a sole source.

If you take a Cambridge meal a half an hour or so before that fourth 400-calorie meal, you will find how little the temptation is to accept any more food.

The drinking of the eight glasses of water each day should continue during this period of semi-dieting. And may water consumption become the splendid habit of a lifetime!

The optimism, the faith, the hope reposed in any diet is that at last here will be that diet of diets. Eureka! Finally, here it is, the perfect diet. Overweight never again.

Immortal last words.

But now, at long, long last, there is a diet that fulfills hopes and answers prayers.

The Cambridge Diet is the initiation into a lifetime of revised eating habits, weight and girth control, and superb nutrition that comes easily and naturally.

Here the Cambridge Diet meshes with the Cambridge Plan.

The Cambridge Plan — like diamonds — is forever.

The underlying assumption of the Cambridge Plan is that no one reverts to gross eating habits, regains lost pounds.

Each individual should discover, by personal experiment, how much food is right for him/her to maintain his/her ideal weight.

Out of the Cambridge Kitchens pour suggestions to aid in this regulatory goal. Suggestions for 800-calorie meals, 600-calorie meals, 400-calorie meals, 200-calorie snacks, 100-calorie snacks, 50-calorie snacks. (Only 50 calories in the Cooked Vegetables Italian, a melange of six vegetables!)

(One Cambridge Group Counselor, a chef manqué, holds a Cambridge buffet once a month. Counselors and those patrons who are no longer dieting sample a Lucullan feast of foods that dazzle the eye and start the taste buds salivating — all to the accompaniment of lovely California wines.)

Having graduated from the Cambridge Diet does not mean we cannot live it up, now and again, all the rest of our lives.

It does not mean we can't have a cocktail or a creme brûlée from time to time.

But here now we have a nutritional safety net.

If a pound or two or three or more comes creeping back, there is such an easy fall-back salvation.

Return to Cambridge as sole nutrition for as long as needs be to get back into fighting fit shape.

As sole source or supplement, the Cambridge Diet can provide a lifetime guarantee for weight maintenance and surpassing nutrition.

15

CAMBRIDGE CUISINE

The following are a sampling of the 400-calorie meals created in the Cambridge Kitchens. It is recommended that any person coming off an extended period of dieting with the Cambridge product meals as the sole source of nutrition do so by adding one 400-calorie meal a day to the three regular Cambridge meals.

POULET A L'ORANGE

(Served with Rice and Broccoli)

Servings: 4

4 chicken breasts—6 oz. raw with bone (5 oz. without bone)
Salt and pepper to taste
1 cup orange juice
2 tsp. grated orange peel
pinch of allspice
¼ tsp. poultry seasoning
1 tbsp. Dijon mustard

Bake chicken breasts in 400° oven about 20 minutes to render fat out of skin. Then combine orange juice, grated rind, allspice, poultry seasoning, and mustard and pour over chicken breasts that have been drained of fat. Continue baking but reduce oven temperature to 350° for another 20–25 minutes or until chicken is done. Baste while cooking. Garnish with slice of orange.

Rice *(½ cup cooked rice per serving)*

Heat 1¼ cups of lightly salted (about ½ teaspoon salt) water in saucepan to boil. Then add ½ cup raw rice, reduce heat, cover, and simmer 15–20 minutes. Cook until all water is absorbed.

Steamed Broccoli

One whole stalk per person. Using a vegetable peeler, trim stalks of tough fiber. Steam broccoli until tender (about 10 minutes) and season to taste.

BEEF STROGANOFF

(Served with Noodles, Lima Beans, and Carrots)

Servings: 4

12 oz. roundsteak, trimmed of all separable fat and cubed
2 small onions (6 oz. total) coarse chopped
2 cups mushrooms (8 oz.) sliced
¼ cup tomato puree
1 cup beef stock
1 cup red wine
¼ cup flour (1 oz.)
1 tsp. thyme
1 bay leaf
1 tsp. savory
1 tsp. salt
¾ cup low-fat yoghurt

Brown the beef and onions in nonstick cookware, using no oil. If such cookware is unavailable, broil the meat. Combine the remaining ingredients except the yoghurt. Simmer gently for at least 2 hours. Place a generous tablespoon of yoghurt on each portion of stroganoff when serving.

Kitchen Hints

Stewing beef may be used if desired. However, it should be as lean as possible and well trimmed of all fat. If canned beef stock is used, add only ½ teaspoon of salt.

Noodles

Cook the noodles in boiling water 8–10 minutes with ½ teaspoon of salt. Drain and serve ½ cup (3 oz.) noodles per portion.

Lima Beans and Carrots

These vegetables may be steamed or boiled (preferably steamed) until they reach the desired texture. One serving consists of ½ cup (3 oz.) of each vegetable. Lima beans cook in about 30 minutes. Carrots cook in 15–20 minutes.

FRITTATA
(Served with Fruit Compote)

Servings: 4

½ cup onion (3 oz.) chopped
⅔ cup mushrooms (2½ oz.) sliced
¼ cup chicken stock or white wine
4 medium eggs
¼ tsp. dried oregano
¼ tsp. nutmeg
low-sodium salt and cayenne pepper to taste
1 cup nonfat milk
1 cup cooked, diced chicken breast (4 oz.) skin and bone removed
1½ cups breadcrumbs
1 cup frozen chopped spinach (7 oz.) defrosted
½ cup low-fat cottage cheese (2½ oz.)

Simmer the onion and mushrooms in the stock or wine until the onion is transparent. Beat the eggs lightly with the seasoning and milk. Combine all the ingredients and pour into a baking dish. Bake in a moderate (350°) oven for 40 minutes, or until a knife inserted in the custard comes out clean.

Fruit Compote

Combine 1 cup fresh orange sections (6 oz.) cut up, 1 cup apple, (3½ oz.) diced and 1 cup banana slices (5 oz.) in a covered dish, reserving some of the orange sections to squeeze over the remaining fruit.

POACHED SOLE JULIENNE

(Served with Potatoes, with Cantaloupe for Dessert)

Servings: 4

1½ lbs. sole filets
2 cups diced tomato (peeled and seeded)
4 oz. leeks, julienned (cut into thin strips)
2 carrots, julienned
2 celery stalks, julienned
1 cup dry white wine
low-sodium salt

Place sole in baking dish and cover with diced tomatoes, julienned leeks, carrots, and celery. Pour in the wine, cover baking dish and bake at 350° approximately 20 to 30 minutes or until tender.

Note: *Each portion of cooked fish should equal 4 oz.*

Potatoes

One steamed or boiled potato per person, seasoned lightly with salt, (or low-sodium substitute) white pepper, and 1 tbsp. chopped parsley. (Potoatoes cook in about 20 minutes.)

Cantaloupe

Sliced cantaloupe, about ½ cup or ¼ of melon.

TUNA SALAD IN A PAPAYA

Serving: 1

1 papaya
5 oz. tuna (low-sodium albacore, packed in water)*
1 tbsp. mayonnaise
1 tsp. Dijon mustard
3 water chestnuts, small dice
1½ oz. snow peas, blanched, julienned on diagonal

*Do not drain.

Cut papaya in half and remove seeds; one portion equals 2 halves. Mix tuna, mayonnaise, mustard, water chestnuts, snow peas together. Fill each half of papaya with salad. Place on lettuce leaves. Garnish each half with blanched whole snow peas. Vanda orchid may be substituted for tomato rose.

COTTAGE PIE

Servings: 4

12 oz. lean ground beef
1 cup onions (4 oz.) chopped
2 cups carrots (8 oz.) sliced
1 cup green peas (4 oz.)
1 cup mushrooms (4 oz.) sliced
2 cups beef stock
1 cup water or ½ cup water or ½ cup water plus ½ cup red wine
Worcestershire sauce (about 1 tsp.)
thyme to taste (about ½ tsp.)
pepper to taste (about ¼ tsp.)

Saute the ground beef and onions until the onions are translucent. Drain well in order to remove all excess fat. Combine with the remaining ingredients and simmer gently until the carrots are tender.

Topping

6 medium (about 24 oz.) potatoes, boiled, drained and mashed. Mix with ½ cup of nonfat milk.

Place the filling in a casserole dish and cover with the mashed potatoes. Place in a moderate oven (350°) for about 20 minutes then serve.

Note: *For best results, use extra lean ground beef (ground round). In this case, 2 teaspoons of butter may be added to the mashed potatoes.*

BREAST OF CHICKEN WITH MUSTARD, LEMON & CAPERS
(Served with Rice Pilaf and Julienne of Carrots)

Servings: 4

4 boned, raw chicken breasts with skin removed (4½ oz. each)
1 cup chicken stock

Sauce

1 tbsp. nonfat milk
1 tbsp. water
1 tbsp. all-purpose white flour
½ tsp. dry mustard
1 tbsp. capers
Juice of ½ medium lemon
Lemon slices for garnish

Chicken

Saute breasts for 10 minutes on each side in a nonstick skillet, or simmer 20 minutes in enough chicken stock plus water or a little white wine to barely cover. Remove to a platter and keep warm.

Sauce

Bring chicken stock and additional poaching liquid, if any, to a boil. Combine flour and mustard, and make a paste by adding milk and water. When the liquid is boiling, stir in the paste, lower the heat to simmer and cook, stir-

ring occasionally, until the flour taste has disappeared, about 20 minutes. Remove from heat. Add the lemon juice and capers. To serve, pour the sauce over the chicken and garnish with lemon slices.

Rice Pilaf *(½ cup pilaf per serving)*

Combine ¾ cup brown rice, ½ cup chopped onions, ½ cup sliced mushrooms, 2 cups chicken stock and ½ teaspoon salt in a saucepan. Bring to a boil. Lower the heat to a simmer and cover. After about 40 minutes, or once the rice is tender, add ½ cup green peas and continue to cook gently for about 5 more minutes.

Julienne Of Carrots

Trim, peel and julienne 4 cups (1 lb.) of carrots and steam or boil in as little water as possible until tender (about 15 minutes). Season with lemon juice, salt (or low-sodium substitute) and, if desired, a pinch of ground cumin.

16

MEDICAL ADVISORY

E*verybody* loses weight on the Cambridge Diet – with astonishing speed.

On 330 calories a day everybody begins consuming for additional energy requirements those stored-up deposits of unwanted unhealthy fat.

The weight losses are comparable to those achievable by going on a total fast.

Individuals have differing rates of metabolism, however, so the rate at which people lose weight varies.

The Cambridge Diet is a balanced very low calorie diet of top quality protein (33 grams per day), carbohydrates (44 grams, including nondigestible carbohydrate for fiber), fat (3 grams), vitamins and minerals and trace elements.

Only in Cambridge has *everything* been added that the body is known to need – and added in proper amounts and proportions – to insure maximum nutrition for up to four weeks. Present also are the electrolytes, which are essential for maintaining the proper acid-base ration in the body and for carrying necessary impulses to body tissues so that they function adequately.

The Cambridge Diet contains 100 percent of everything else but only 75 percent of the recommended daily allowance of protein. Dr. Howard and his team discovered that with the reduction of calories — and the carbohydrate balance — that was more than sufficient protein to prevent any loss of nitrogen equilibrium. (In general, most people consume more protein than they need.) The body consumes fat, not lean tissue.

Diabetics can flourish on the Cambridge Diet. Along with the weight loss and superlative nutrition, many of them are able to reduce their medication — and the health risks associated with diabetes. There have been no metabolic or clinical complications or abnormalities in cardiac function, as evaluated by electrocardiogram, with diabetes patients.

People with high blood pressure are well advised to go on the diet. The sodium content is low (1,500mg. of sodium per day), and the weight reduction can only be a boon to hypertension. But if on medication, prospective dieters should first get clearance from their physicians.

Hypoglycemics may respond favorably to the Cambridge Diet; many find that both their physical and emotional states show remarkable improvement. Some prefer to take six "minimeals" rather than three full Cambridge meals in order to help maintain an even blood glucose level.

Diabetics, hypertensives, hypoglycemics and others with medical problems should use Cambridge only under a physician's guidance.

Serum cholesterol and triglyceride levels are reduced, on the average, by 21 and 45 percent, respectively, on this diet.

It is urged that no one use diuretics on this diet unless directed to by a physician; the body could be depleted of essential potassium.

No amphetamines either; the diet has a natural faculty for lowering the appetite and the craving for food.

No dieter should go on the Cambridge Diet as a sole source of nutrition for more than 28 consecutive days. If further weight losses are indicated to achieve desired goals, then have a week or so when the three Cambridge meals are supplemented by an additional 400-calorie meal before resuming Cambridge as sole source.

You must drink eight or more glasses of water a day; the intake of water insures the proper functioning of the kidneys and helps flush out the "ashes" of burned-up fat.

Other noncaloric beverages are permitted, but it is best to go easy on diet sodas because of their sodium content – and on caffeinated drinks because they tend to jangle the nervous system.

Alcoholic beverages are stictly verboten; not only do they contain calories but they cause water retention and bloating.

Any side effects should be minimal and momentary. In the words of Deor's Lament, "This too shall pass." And quickly.

There have been no serious medical complications that have occurred when the Cambridge Diet is taken as directed.

Listen to your body. If you are really feeling lightheaded or hungry in that first day or two, take a little solid food. But make it something good. Carrot sticks. Unsalted, unbuttered popcorn. A few raw nuts. A banana or an apple. (How magnificent natural food tastes as we become weaned away from lifeless, chemical-ridden food!)

Children can be given the Cambridge Diet as a supplement to their meals; it is impossible to conceive of a better "snack."

Eat each meal immediately or seal it in an airtight container to prevent vitamin loss.

The recommended shelf life for the Cambridge Diet product is 18 months, unopened; three to four months opened, but sealed with the plastic lid. Certain nutrients are rapidly oxidized when in contact with light, air, and heat. The most harmful effects to the product can come from leaving the lid off the can.

Do not do anything with the formula except put it into hot or cold water. Do not boil, bake, or put it into a microwave oven.

Men and women on the Cambridge Diet routinely go about their business; for most there is no need for "taking it easy."

Exercise can only go hand in glove with any weight reduction program, expediting its progress – and ideally should be a part of everyone's daily regimen – but with or without exercise, everyone will rapidly lose weight on the Cambridge Diet.

Some people take so well to the restrictive caloric content of the diet that they ask if it's all right to have just two Cambridge meals a day. No, that isn't all right because the three meals are required to meet the day's nutritional requirements.

There may occur what is called "plateauing," a condition in which no weight losses are registering on the scales. This may be due to water retention and is illusory. The reality is that *progress is being made every day.*

The Cambridge Diet is as safe as it is dynamic.

For his nutritional breakthrough, Dr. Alan N. Howard deserves to be recognized and to be awarded a Nobel Prize in biochemistry.

To quote William M. Helvey, M.D., the Medical Director of The Cambridge Plan International, "The Cambridge Diet Plan is an outstanding advance in medicine that can have a significant impact on the health of the nation. Obesity is a major contributor to heart disease and other serious ailments such as diabetes and hypertension. As with any innovation, there is always a time lag between its introduction and its routine application and acceptance as common knowledge."

17

LISTEN TO THE DOCTORS!

Increasingly members of the medical profession are finding Cambridge to be a safe very low calorie diet that delivers on its promises.

"I have been overweight for most of my life," confides Dr. Bill M. Escoffery of Homestead, Florida, "and was in a pretty sorry state with a gout attack after one of my many fad diets, when my secretary brought a can of the Cambridge Diet into the office and said, 'Here's your answer.'

"In a month I lost the 24 pounds I had always been trying to lose. The gout and related hyperuricemia went away. My blood lipids were the lowest of any patient that I had ever had.

"I lost all the inches I wanted to lose, and I really looked good. Of course, I tried to keep it all a secret. Patients would come in and not recognize me. So I finally had to come out of the closet about the Cambridge Diet.

"I'm not the only doctor in our family. My father is a retired family practitioner, and he and my mother are on the Cambridge Diet. So is my brother, who is an ophthalmologist, and my brother-in-law, an orthopedic surgeon. It all stems from my success and my medical reports which establish the credibility of the diet.

"With my own overweight patients, without exception, unless there is some very, very unusual medical circumstance, they are put on the Cambridge Diet. I monitor them and keep a record of their weight and blood pressure and measure them. I also adjust the medication of those who have been on diuretic or blood pressure medicine. I have found nothing in my years of medical practice that compares with the Cambridge Diet."

Dr. Anthony A. Conte of Beaver, Pennsylvania, a prominent bariatric physician, says, "In my practice, the Cambridge Diet has helped me instill confidence because, taken as directed, the patients have had a substantial weight loss week after week. They were more energetic, experienced little or no hunger, held to their motivation, experienced desirable health changes, such as lowering of high blood pressure and their cholesterol and triglycerides levels returning to normal. The simplicity of use and the palatability of the Cambridge Diet, plus the excellent results, help prevent 'diet drop-out.'"

Dr. Conte goes on to observe astutely, "Unfortunately, a lot of doctors in this country are not familiar with the Cambridge Plan, and they confuse it with the liquid protein diet."

Before their conversion, doctors confess their initial skepticism.

"As a family physician with my own medical center and as a former chief of staff of a hospital," discloses Glenn M. Doornink, M.D. of Wapato, Washington, a Fellow of the American Academy of Family Physicians, "I was initially skeptical about the Cambridge Diet and was hesitant to recommend its use to those patients who approached me wanting my permission to start the diet. Finally my son, who was then a resident physician in Internal Medicine and had been introduced to the use of the Cambridge Diet while in training with a local cardiologist, convinced me that he was really pleased with the documented research and the contents of the formula.

"After careful examination of the plan and the more recent research done, I myself decided to give Cambridge the ultimate test and try it myself. I subsequently lost 50 pounds using the Cambridge Diet and not only our friends and neighbors but physicians began asking me about my success.

"It was easy to share information about the Cambridge Diet with other physicians because of the clinical research and documentation that I discovered in my reading. Not only did other physicians in my community start recommending the diet plan to their patients, but some of them referred certain patients to me for counselling.

"I am excited (and so are my patients) with this newly discovered method of controlling these conditions that are often frustrating to manage, namely overweight, hypertension, and diabetes. My patients now find that they can control their weight easily and inexpensively with the helpful support of their physicians, their Cambridge Counselor, and their Cambridge friends."

Declares Stephen N. Kreitzman, Ph.D., Director, Center for Nutrition and Dental Health, Emory University, Atlanta, Georgia: "The Cambridge Diet is based upon sound nutrition principles which have been extensively researched for over half a century. Formula diets are in common usage for human health maintenance throughout the world and are well recognized to provide for good nutrition. The specific formula researched by Dr. Howard and others has been studied for more than a decade for the purpose of weight reduction and in my experience, both as a nutrition scientist and as a weight control subject it has deomonstrated both safety and effectiveness. As part of a pilot study at Emory University I have used the product for a personal loss of 103 pounds at this writing. Other subjects in my pilot study have lost more than 70 pounds each; one of these individuals was my wife who is a professional chef, restaurant reviewer and food writer."

Leopold S. Kaplan, M.D., of Edison, New Jersey, was skeptical too, but he decided to attend a Cambridge meeting with his wife after hearing other people talking about their success with the plan. He went on the weight-loss program and lost 16 pounds in 18 days and felt better and better each day—hadn't felt so well in 25 years!

"My wife and I must have started 200 people on Cambridge and have gotten people in the medical community involved as well," declares Dr. Kaplan. "The most uniform effect that people seem to have while taking Cambridge is that they feel great and have more energy. A typical example of a Cambridge experience is the wife who says she now has a new husband because he lost 80 pounds in eight weeks using the Cambridge weight loss program. I just thank God Cambridge came along."

James Howenstine M.D., of San Francisco, first heard of the Cambridge Diet by sitting next to someone on a plane who said he had lost 40 pounds in 50 days and felt great and hadn't been hungry. This revelation was baffling, if true, inasmuch as Dr. Howenstine had never had good results treating obesity in his medical practice. He read the literature on Dr. Howard's work and decided to try it for himself.

"I was surprised how easy it was," marvels Dr. Howenstine. "I lost 15 pounds in ten days and 28 pounds in 21 days, and I have maintained this loss.

"My own results encouraged me to recommend the diet to my patients who were struggling with a weight problem, either large or small, and those who have gone on the diet faithfully have all lost weight. Many have reached their goal weight."

Francis J. Cinelli, D.O. of Bangor, Pennsylvania, finds that 40 percent of his practice is weight control, and he tries to educate his patients about the risk factor that is involved with being overweight.

"But I've had my own overweight problems," reveals Dr. Cinelli, "which various diets have solved only temporarily. Then in June of 1982 I tried the Cambridge Diet. You don't know how a product works until you try it, and I wanted to try the Cambridge Diet myself before recommending it to my patients. And it worked rapidly and effectively. I lost 30 pounds in four weeks and felt great with a high energy level. I feel that the Cambridge Diet is the sensible nondrug way to lose weight and keep it off, and I recommend it to my patients."

"My area of specialization is occupational and preventive medicine," explains Ronald F. Sorenson, M.D., of Madison, Connecticut, medical director with a large aircraft corporation.

"One of the best attributes of the Cambridge plan is its ease and versatility in providing assured adequate basic daily nutrition, coupled with the freedom from worry and concern regarding one's nutritional intake. The truly impressive results I find in my patients and others using the Cambridge is the ability it provides for people to finally be in control of their nutrition and weight. They look better and feel better, leading to improved self-image and the loss of guilt normally associated with being overweight.

"I think more and more physicians are becoming aware of the benefits of Cambridge, not only for people who need to lose weight but for the nutritional needs it fulfills."

Richard Anonsen, M.D., Minneapolis: "In my practice, I have used the Cambridge Diet on my overweight patients and have monitored them regularly.

"I have noticed a marked reduction in cholesterol and triglyceride levels consistently among the patients who use the Cambridge Diet, and I've taken some diabetics off their insulin, some hypertensive patients off their high blood pressure medication.

"The results have been excellent, and people feel good while on the diet, which is important. I've lost ten pounds myself, and now I take it for the nutritional benefit."

George A. Bray, M.D., Los Angeles: "Not to be confused with the liquid protein diets, the diet developed by Dr. Alan N. Howard and his colleagues in Cambridge and London, England, has used high quality proteins. There is nothing apparent in this formulation which should be in any way harmful or deleterious when used according to the direction."

R. H. Richardson, D.P.M., a Grand Junction, Colorado, podiatrist: "Before I discovered the Cambridge Diet, I was counting the nails in my coffin. My blood sugar count was 361. I had eleven point five uric acid, and I was in bad shape. I was so convinced I was going to die, I took a whole load of my clothes down to the Salvation Army—and it took three of us to carry them all in.

"I simply could not get a handle on my weight problem. I was eating maybe four to six thousand calories a day. Then I found out about the Cambridge diet from a pharmaceutical representative who had been calling on me for years. Within 24 hours I was on it—and losing weight.

"I admit to being over 270, and I didn't keep track of how fast I lost. But I had a tailor come in and alter my clothes as I was losing, and I know that by the time the clothes were ready for me in a week, they were already too big.

"I looked so different, patients would come in my office and walk right by me and ask the receptionist who the new doctor was. That's a real boost!"

Let's hear too from Arlene Davis of North Miami Beach, Florida, who is an Advanced Registered Nurse Practitioner and Assistant Professor of Nursing at a community college:

"I'm really impressed with the eight and a half years of research that went into the development of the Cambridge Diet. With its balanced nutrition and 100 percent of the U.S. RDA of vitamins and minerals, I feel comfortable using it myself and recommending it to my associates."

18

CAMBRIDGE, THE BREAKFAST-LUNCH-DINNER OF CHAMPIONS

This sporting society we live in!

This sporting society is in blissful collusion with the world of Cambridge.

Everywhere trainers and team physicians and coaches who must look after the well-being of athletes are putting those athletes on the Cambridge Diet to insure that their nutrition is top notch.

Ex-professional athletes who find that it's too easy to get out of shape once the playing days are over discover that Cambridge can return them quickly to their peaks of prowess.

Let's go to the record and hear directly from some of the men themselves.

"The Cambridge Nutrition Plan is truly a product that is ahead of its time", avers Otho Davis, head trainer of the Philadelphia Eagles. "The perfectly balanced formula which includes all the vitamins, minerals and nutrients, plus trace elements and electrolytes, insures me that our athletes are getting all the proper nutrition, which is so hard to get in professional athletes' busy schedules.

"The amazing thing is that it is only 330 calories so if needed it can help the athlete stay trim. It is a good year-round program, and I am pleased with the results. It can be an asset to any sports program."

Here's what Joe Klecko, defensive lineman of the New York Jets, has to say:

"Being a defensive lineman, I've never had a weight problem; in fact, I need to keep my weight up. I put in a very strenuous day, because I'm a big weight-lifter along with my football practices and regular season play. I've been on all kinds of protein diets and vitamin supplements to keep my nutrition level up, but when we started keeping the Cambridge Diet in our training room, I noticed a big change. I started taking Cambridge in the mornings before I work out and then afterward, and before lifting weights, in addition to my regular meals.

"I was surprised at the results. I noticed in my workouts that I wasn't tiring at all, and even after a long day of practicing, running, and lifting weights that can be tiring, I still had energy. I just kept on going. Now I take Cambridge three or four times a day just to keep up the high energy level Cambridge has given me. I think it's great!"

Charles Hodgson, coach for the men's swimming team, University of Miami, comments, "I went on the Cambridge Diet and told my swimming club I would lose 15 pounds in two weeks to show how easy it was, and ended up losing 17 pounds in two weeks! You know what? Those were the most efficient two weeks of my life. I slept only five hours a night and awoke with boundless energy.

"That's what stimulated my interest in using Cambridge for my swimmers. I was looking for something for athletes to use to lose weight and still be able to train, and since then I have had great success using it this way. One girl who was a good swimmer but had always been overweight went on the weight-loss plan and lost about 20 pounds. Since that time, about a year ago, she has kept it off and she has been improving her 'time' constantly; more importantly, it's changed her whole self image.

"For the men's team, I feel the nutritional balance of Cambridge is important, and boy, do they seem to go through my supply quickly! The body fat ratio of all my swimmers is consistently good now, and I think they are just healthier; you know college kids don't eat well. All you can get in the cafeteria lines is carbohydrates and overcooked foods devoid of nutrients. I have found Cambridge is great for athletes who tend to get nervous."

Bob Reese, head athletic trainer with the New York Jets, shares with us this information: "During the training camp period we made the Cambridge Diet available for everyone, and I would counsel individuals as they requested it or as they used it. I find that with the Cambridge Diet three times a day, it certainly does not take as much regular food to give me a full feeling.

"It's so difficult when you get into high pressure situations to keep track of what you eat, because diet is the last thing you worry about. That's one good thing about having the Cambridge Diet around, as far as keeping up your nutritional balance. Having it available here in the locker room, the players have been making some up, and I tell them to make some up for me, and I get my nutrition that way because we rarely break for lunch."

"I have worked for many years with young athletes of all ages and their trainers striving toward the peak of physical fitness and well-being," we are told by Gene Felker, chairman of the board, National Football Clinics.

"A year ago, my physician advised me to try the Cambridge Diet and said he would monitor my weight-loss progress. I started the diet on February 15, 1982, with the goal of getting back to my ideal 193 pounds college weight. I proceeded to reach this goal quickly and safely, losing a total of 40 pounds, eliminating those problems that had accompanied my overweight condition, and have taken three Cambridge meals per day ever since then to maintain the goal weight and high energy level I had achieved.

"I have shared the Cambridge Diet with hundreds of friends and athletic associates so that they too could derive the same tremendous nutritional benefits from this simple, easy-to-use formula."

Jeff Mitchell, of Ellicott City, Maryland, who is "Mr. Maryland, Tall Class of 1982," says, "When body-builders prepare for a contest, we have to do 'skin down', which means that we have to get rid of all the body fat that we possibly can so that muscle striation shows through the skin.

"By using the Cambridge Diet when we train, we get the vitamins and minerals our bodies need, in balance, while we're reducing the fat but maintaining the muscle size and also maintaining our good health.

"Bob Magersupp and Lisl D. Dutterer, who recently won the 1982 U.S. Classic Couples Body-Building Championships, used the Cambridge Diet during training to help give them that extra special trim, firm, toned appearance that made the difference."

Dennis Franks, former center for the Philadelphia Eagles and Detroit Lions, observes, "For my position as center, when you weigh 270 pounds, that's what you're paid for. My profession was to move people for a living.

The problem was when I stopped playing, I didn't stop eating the huge quantities of food I had needed on the football field. As a businessman behind a desk, my 275 pounds was uncomfortable, unattractive, and unprofessional.

"In April of 1981, I started the Cambridge Diet and lost 14 pounds in three days and 42 pounds in three-and-a-half weeks. I still get up every morning at five-thirty to go train. I run an average of two miles and then do an hour of Olympic weight lifting. I really believe the reason I do so well and get so much done in a day is because of Cambridge.

"According to the NFL statistics, the average life span for an offensive lineman is age 55 because they normally do not lose the weight after they're done playing, and the muscles turn to fat, and that puts a strain on the heart. I knew that, and I wanted to be sure I didn't follow that path. I wanted to live longer than 55. And now, with Cambridge three times a day, I have this feeling I'll be a good 75."

Dave Schultz, a professional hockey player (member of the Stanley Cup Champion Philadelphia Flyers of 1974 and 1975), has this to say: "I made a promise to myself never to go up to 200 pounds again after I stopped playing professional hockey. I hated dieting, but I had never had to worry about it before. So I tried a couple of diets, but I felt terrible. I'd lose the five pounds or so I wanted to lose, and then I'd gain them right back.

"Then I heard about the Cambridge Diet. I went from 205 to 194 in less than a week, and then I lost another four pounds, to get down to 190, which is an excellent weight for me since I'm six feet one inch. That's less than my playing weight and I feel great." (Would that Dave had known about Cambridge during his pre-hockey days when the nutritional benefits would have helped him so much!)

Wally Hilgenberg was starting linebacker in all four Super Bowls that the Minnesota Vikings have played in and was a regular for the Vikings and the Detroit Lions during his 16-year career in professional football.

Wally: "But after being out of football for two years, even after dieting, working out, playing racquetball, and running on a regular basis, the lightest I could get was about 221. On Cambridge I dropped from 221 to 210 pounds. I was totally amazed at what happened and how good I felt.

"Then I went on a five-day fishing trip into Canada, with pancakes for breakfast, shore lunches, eating everything in sight. And I came back home with the fear that everything I had accomplished in those first four days would have been destroyed, but to my surprise, I'd gained back only two and a half pounds. I went back on the Cambridge Diet, and two weeks later

I'd lost a total of 23 pounds and was down to 198, two pounds lower than my goal. That was eight months ago, and I have not gained back a pound.

"But the thing that really impressed me was that I had come to a point where working out caused everything to ache—my ankles, my knees, even my hamstrings. But now that I am on Cambridge I no longer have any joint pain or muscle pain—I feel great—I can work out three times a week, and I don't get sore. I think it is from proper, balanced nutrition."

Wayne Glusker, 50 kilometer racewalker, National Track and Field Team, U.S. World Cup Track and Field Team: "I have access to a lot of free nutritional supplements and vitamins, but I've stopped taking them now that I have found the Cambridge Diet.

"With the Cambridge Diet as a nutritional supplement, I know I am getting the balance and the nutrients I need. My energy level is much higher than it ever was before, and I need much less sleep, and my chronic back problems have cleared up after being on Cambridge for about ten weeks. When I am training hard, I need a lot of endurance because I put in a lot of miles, 20 a day before I go to my eight-hour-a-day job. The Cambridge formula really helps me overcome fatigue."

"After I retired from playing football with the Philadelphia Eagles," recalls the sports director of WFIL-AM Philadelphia, Vince Papale, "I put on a few extra pounds that I couldn't get off no matter what I did. A friend recommended the Cambridge Diet, and I lost the weight I wanted to lose almost immediately—within a week and a half or so, I shed 13 pounds, which got me back down to my playing weight, which was 198. But it was so easy and so fast, I decided to go down to 190, the weight I'd been in college. And I did that in another week.

"I feel great and keep getting all kinds of compliments from people who say that I look like I'm in shape to play ball again.

"With my radio job, I get up at four-thirty A.M. and am in my office by five-thirty to go on the air at six for the morning commute. Then I'm back on the air during the evening drive, and I do pregame shows for the Seventy-sixers. It's a busy schedule, an easy 14-hour day for me. But with Cambridge three times a day, I never run out of energy. I have my three Cambridge meals and one light meal a day and have no trouble maintaining my weight. I feel like I'm in really good nutritional balance."

Another Pennsylvanian, Bill Bergey of Chadds Ford, a former All-Pro Middle Linebacker, shares *his* experience with us: "After playing pro football for 13 years and never having a weight problem, I figured that I deserved a break. I wasn't going to exercise—I was just going to let Mother

Nature heal my body from the bruising I had taken over the years. But then I started gaining weight up to 250, then 260. When I hit 269¾ I told myself something had to be done. So I started on the Cambridge Diet. And in 52 days I'd lost 48 pounds.

"The Cambridge Diet gave me everything I needed—I had the pep, I had the vigor, and I really felt great...I'm on the banquet circuit a lot, and I've found that people really respect you when you're on a diet. There are some who say they can't diet because they're always having food put in front of them. But I don't really find that to be true at all. I threw away all my fat, fatter, and fattest clothes and bought myself a new wardrobe."

Since 1960, Bill Babcock, a 44 year-old instructor at Anchorage Community College, in Alaska has been leading mountain-climbing expeditions to South America (specifically to some fifty peaks over 17,000 feet in Venezuela, Colombia, Ecuador, Peru, and Bolivia.) Over the years, he had been plagued with the problem of climbers losing strength at the higher altitudes, with the concomitant risk of pulmonary edema.

Hearing about Cambridge in the autumn of 1982, Mr. Babcock decided to give it a two week try before departing once again for Ecuador. There the extended trek to El Altar covered twenty miles of difficult trail, followed by a hike from 9,000 to 15,000 feet. During these extreme exertions, Bill kept on using the Cambridge Diet as a supplement, and he reports enthusiastically: "The result for me was simply amazing! Other members of of our party felt very ill and suffered from headaches and vomiting. At no time did I suffer these same problems. The entire time I felt strong and very healthy, and, even carrying very heavy loads for hours on end, I did not appear to be exhausted at the end of the day. Apparently, an additional benefit of the program was my feeling of well-being mentally. Many climbers feel that the mental factor is what really gets people up mountains and pulls them through in survival situations. I felt that the Cambridge Program has this added benefit in that one appears to keep his mental capacities at a fine tune through regular use of the product."

You could hear similar accolades from a hundred thousand or so other great sports.

Listen, if Cambridge is perfect enough for these terrific guys whose careers depend upon their keeping themselves in tippy-top physical shape...

19

LOVE (OF CAMBRIDGE) HAS MANY FACES

How do we love thee, Cambridge? Let us count the ways.

The Cambridge Diet is so adaptable that it fits into many peoples' lives—embellishes them—in so many different ways.

"I loved Cambridge from my very first sip!" exclaims the beautiful actress Meredith MacRae. "I've been traveling a lot lately for NBC's *Fantasy.* More often than not, my call to start work is five A.M. and room service is never open, so I just put some Cambridge in a glass, add water, mix it up, and I'm all set to start the day. My favorite is chocolate. I add three frozen strawberries and ice. Cambridge is the greatest!"

"I want to lose ten more pounds before production starts," says TV and film star James Brolin in reference to a forthcoming television series. "And it's good to know it's not going to take all the willpower in the world to do it. Cambridge is the most convenient source of nutrition I have been able to find. I don't have to go to all the trouble and expense of trying to put together all the various nutritional elements my body needs to be at its best."

Highly energized Helen Nirva, an instructor of the mentally retarded at the Fergus Falls (Minnesota) State Hospital, tells us, "I take Cambridge for breakfast and for lunch and go like a house on fire all day long and have a terrific dinner. I haven't put one pound back on since I lost those 20 pounds a year ago when I first when on Cambridge."

Actor Patrick O'Neal takes along his Cambridge shaker when he travels — and takes it into some of the fancy restaurants where they think he's crazy, but that doesn't throw him.

"From being in fairly good trim to start with," explains O'Neal, "by using the Cambridge Diet I've been able to go to an extra level, a level I haven't been at since high school. Every time I turn around I have to have my clothes taken in. I went from feeling okay to feeling extremely well, which surprised me.... It's a lovely experience."

Yes, and Cambridge can be the conduit to love as well as the object of it.

"David and I met at our Cambridge Counselor's home," confides Janice Horne of Knoxville, Tennessee. "Three weeks later we knew we were in love, and three months later we were married. On our wedding day, we not only celebrated our marriage but our combined weight loss of 222 pounds on the Cambridge Diet Plan. I wore a beautiful size six wedding dress instead of a 22½ dress I needed when I weighed 243 pounds. David was so handsome in his size 44 suit instead of the 56 extra large he needed at 331 pounds."

New York Post editorial cartoonist Paul Rigby who at 58 had the goal — and succeeded at it — of making himself fit enough to play in a World Squash Classic, recalls: "I used to be somewhat muscle bound, very tense through the shoulders and that sort of thing, but now that I've been on the Cambridge Diet, I notice that this muscular tension that I've had for years, seems to have dropped away. I can run around the squash court more quickly, and I'm much more relaxed in all departments, sexually as well as athletically. I feel more energetic, more mentally alert, and I'm doing everything a little better. My wife Marlene says that even my cartoons have improved!"

Opera singer Evelyn Ronell dispels a myth about opera singers:

"The fear is that if they diet, they will lose their voice. I'm a soprano, and my voice is better than ever since I went on the Cambridge Diet and lost 22 pounds easily and quickly. Ordinarily, if I diet, the first place I lost weight is my face. Not so with Cambridge. My face looks lovely, and the fat came off the rest of my body where I needed to lose, so that looks lovely now, too. On other diets, whenever I reached a certain point, I would get sick or have a sore throat or would go promptly right back up again. With Cambridge I passed that set point with flying colors. I'm down to 105 pounds now, and I feel very alive, very peppy, and very happy."

Peppy? Down New Mexico way there's a sexagenarian charmer —

Eleanor Philpott of Albuquerque—who went on the Cambridge Diet primarily for nutrition.

"I have spent thousands of dollars on nutritionists, M.D.s, clinics, quacks, medication, and supplements," she laments. "Balanced nutrition is the answer. I am dedicated always to use the Cambridge Diet. It has been a miracle to me since I am now able to enjoy life. Now I have a great deal of energy."

Jim Timberlake is editor of *The Daily Digest of the U.S. Senate* and puts in some very long days, particularly at the end of the Congressional session.

Last summer Jim went on the Cambridge Diet and lost a total of 64 pounds and comments, "This year is the first year for as far back as I can remember that I didn't get sick by the time the session was over. I didn't get any colds. I didn't have the flu, and I attribute that to Cambridge. I think I'm healthier for it. I know that many senators and members of Congress have come to rely on the Cambridge Diet to help maintain their weight and energy, too."

Claude O'Donovan of McMinnville, Oregon, talks about the amazing change his son underwent when he started taking Cambridge:

"Lance used to consume enormous amounts of sugar—he would sit down with a two-liter bottle of Pepsi and down it in one swig! He also was a very hyperactive, abrasive young man, whose temperament had almost alienated him from society. He couldn't show affection to us, his parents, either. We had tried to encourage him to take Cambridge but he refused. Then one day he needed a part for his car, (he had just started driving) and came to me.

"I struck a bargain with him that I would help him out if he would agree to start taking Cambridge three times a day. He became angry but eventually agreed, and within two days of taking Cambridge faithfully, we had a different son. For the first time in years Lance wasn't craving so many sweets and—most important of all—he started showing affection for Karen and me. Then everyone started noticing the change in his personality: his teachers, friends, etc....By the way, our daugther also takes Cambridge, along with her meals, because not only can she keep her figure trim, but it also keeps her skin clear! It's a wonderful family experience all the way around."

As an economist with the Bureau of Economics of the Federal Trade Commission, Ed Manfield is on the Washington scene too. But he is also an International Master and World Class Bridge Expert who competes all over the globe in World Bridge Championships. In October of 1982 he went to Biarritz, where the bridge playing was also an endurance contest that at one point went for 20 straight hours.

"I used the Cambridge Diet as my sole source of nutrition for the entire tournament," said Ed. "I find that Cambridge is excellent for me during bridge tournaments because it's important that I'm always mentally alert, that my reflexes and my mind are very sharp. And I find that after an ordinary lunch or dinner, my mind just isn't as quick as after I've had Cambridge. Cambridge makes me more alert and gives me more energy and stamina, which is a big advantage. Besides that, while other competitors are spending time hunting for restaurants around town, I can spend that time relaxing in between sessions."

Working people in particular do appreciate this serendipity of found time. The lunch hour becomes an opportunity for doing things—shopping, exercise, taking a book to the park. Not to mention avoiding the expense and aggravation of crowded restaurants.

Now here's a woman—Phyllis Beauvais, Ph.D., by name and distinction, of Roxbury, Connecticut—who had been awarded the demanding role of Titania, the fairy queen, in the local little theater's production of *A Midsummer Night's Dream*. "Who wants to be a 'fat fairy'?" wondered she. Who, indeed? Cambridge to the rescue—our Titania had dropped 23 nasties posthaste before curtain time.

(In real life Phyllis Beauvais and her husband are psychotherapists who deal every day with the emotional problems related to being overweight and think the Cambridge Diet will help "these patients where other diets have failed because enjoying Cambridge is like having a strawberry milk shake or a root beer float. That's not deprivation—that's pleasure!")

"We use the Cambridge Diet in our work with people who have psychological or emotional problems," stress counselors Kenneth Magner, Ph.D., and Jeanadele Magner, Ph.D., of Longwood, Florida, inform us. "The thing we sense almost immediately is an air of well-being with any person in almost any area who takes Cambridge seriously three times a day. They achieve that nutritional balance, even if there's not weight challenge. There's a sense of elation when they see something is going right all of a sudden in their lives. Their bodies are doing something right by them. You really feel this very keenly."

Country singer-songwriter-actor Merle Kilgore had to audition to play *himself* on the NBC-TV special *Living Proof*, the life story of Hank Williams, Jr., with Richard Thomas playing Hank. He knew he had to lose

30 pounds — but fast — because the story goes back about 17 years, when Merle was that much younger and a lot thinner. He heard about the Cambridge Diet from Hank's aunt in Texas who has lost 60 pounds; he went on it; he dropped the pounds and got the part!

"A lot of people think the entertainment business is just a glamour job, but it's really hard work — 24 hours a day," Merle sets the record straight. "We eat at all kinds of odd hours and eat the wrong kind of food, usually after a show, and then go to bed, which is the worst thing you can do.

"The Cambridge Diet really suits my kind of life because it's something I can live with on the road. With other diets you have to have special kinds of foods, and you can't get that in a truck stop or a cafe or a hotel restaurant. Just about everybody in the band is using Cambridge. Half the musicians at the studio where I record in Nashville are on it. They take a Cambridge break now instead of a hot dog break."

Stephanie Zimbalist, who plays Laura Holt in the NBC television series *Remington Steele,* makes this observation: "Working in a television series means a very busy schedule. I have to pace myself and discipline myself to maintain good health. And, because the camera adds ten pounds to your weight, it's a constant battle with the bulge.

"Personally, the Cambridge Diet is great for me. It knocked off those pounds I've always played with. One thing I found remarkable about the Cambridge Diet is that I was not hungry. On the set I'm around food all the time, and yet it doesn't tempt me. I found the diet effortless. It didn't upset my system, and it energized me and got me on a stabilized weight-loss program."

Stephanie's sister, Nancy Zimbalist, who lost 33 pounds she had otherwise been unable to shake, says, "As part of my job, I participate in trade shows all over the country, and I always take my Cambridge Diet and shaker mug with me. I'm never without my Cambridge, never! I've even gotten out of bed at midnight because I've forgotten to have my third Cambridge that day. I'm going on a Carribean vacation soon, so I'm back on the Cambridge Diet sole source to lose a few more pounds so I'll look really fantastic in my bikini!"

Vana Tribbey and Paul Tinder met while doing the television daytime soap, *Another World.* Some months later they were driving cross-country from California to New York, and Vana felt that her metabolism was going out of kilter and she was picking up "saddlebags" from all the sitting in the car and catch-as-catch-can eating. It was a San Antonio manicurist, to whom she complained about the mounting pounds, who gave her a can of the Cambridge Diet. Presto! Within four days she had gone from size seven to size five—eventually to four—and the saddlebags had melted away.

"Paul uses Cambridge as a nutritional supplement and has had wonderful success with it," remarks Vana. "He has always been very athletic, and when he received a severe foot injury (doing a football sequence in the *Magnum P.I.* series) it put him out of commission for several months. He started cutting back on his calories and became impossible to live with. I put him on three Cambridge drinks daily, in addition to his meals, and in a week his disposition was back to normal, and he started losing stored fat and maintaining his lean muscle tissue, which is so important."

Ken Wright, flight crew scheduler for Trans World Airlines, recalls the pilot who came into the scheduling office so trimmed down he didn't recognize him. That's how Ken got introduced to the Cambridge Diet and dropped 50 pounds, which have remained dropped.

"My daughter went on the weight loss program with me and has lost about thirty pounds and has the wonderful side effect of finally being able to eliminate the allergy shots she had taken ever since she was a toddler," Ken discloses. "My wife and son take Cambridge also as a nutritional supplement and my son's hypertension problem seems to have settled down a bit.

"Most people I work with are now taking Cambridge, either for nutrition or weight loss or both. Pilots are always very conscious of being their best and most alert when flying, and those periodic physicals they go through are tough! The stewardesses of course, have to keep their weight under a certain limit; but the list also includes ramp people, security people, office workers—just everyone!"

Nancy Haslett reflects upon her experience as a Playboy Bunny: "We have monthly weigh-ins, and if you're overweight, you don't work. I had tried all sorts of diets, including my own invention of tunafish and vegetables, but I always gained the weight right back.

"With the Cambridge Diet, I lost nine pounds in five days. And the fat just melted off my hips and thighs.... I worked nights from nine P.M. until four in the morning, and we had only half an hour break for dinner. Mixing up a Cambridge formula was so easy—and it really gave me the energy to get through the crazy hours I was working. And I required much less sleep."

Actress Lorna Luft: "The Cambridge Diet is the only diet that has ever really worked for me. I don't like to go on diets where you have to measure everything you eat.

"I lost a lot of weight, very fast, and I lost where I wanted to lose. I started out with the idea of taking off only ten pounds, but they disappeared so quickly and easily that I took off 20, every extra ounce that had been bugging me.

"I'm continuing to use the Cambridge Diet three times a day. I have a lot more energy and feel a lot better, too. I even take it with me on the set when I know I can't get home to eat. Everyone makes jokes that my life revolves around a blender.

"I've turned a lot of people on to the Cambridge Diet. Some of them have lost 17 pounds in only 14 days. They're finding it really works for them, just like it really works for me."

Actor Bob Doran: "Whether you are pursuing a career in films, on stage or television, your appearance is crucial. That's why I decided to drop 31 pounds that I had gained three years ago after I quit smoking. An actress friend told me about the Cambridge Diet, so I decided to try it and found that it was wonderful. I lost 15 pounds in ten days and 23 pounds in 23 days. I also found that I had a tremendous amount of energy, starting around the fourth day. Now I like what I see in the mirror because I see a person with new self-esteem and self-confidence.

"I take Cambridge three times a day and have maintained my weight, and I find that the good news about the Cambridge Diet is really spreading through the acting community."

A stewardess with an international airline: "On a five-day trip between Paris and Tel Aviv I lost eight pounds on the Cambridge Diet. The crew saw the weight coming off right before their eyes and they were amazed. I eventually went from a size ten to a size six uniform.

"My job is very demanding both physically and mentally, so I'm very nutrition conscious. I think whenever you feel run down, you can be subject to depressions and fatigue; and when you're flying and have the responsibility for so many people, it's important to keep up your body for the sake of your mind. I take Cambridge with me on all my flights, and I always find that at least one other member of the crew is on Cambridge too."

The testimonials flow on and on and on, like the Yangtze River. Ad infinitum.

For Cambridge, panegyrics without end.

So many lives being touched, lightened, lifted, gilded, and bonded to other lives!

20

NUTRITIONAL INFORMATION ON THE CAMBRIDGE DIET

Meal size (1 serving) is
1 level scoop . . . . 33.5 grams
Three meals (3 servings) . . . . 100.5 grams
Servings per container 21

	Per Meal	Per Day (3 Meals)
Calories	110	330
Protein	11 grams	33 grams
Carbohydrates	15 grams	44 grams
Fat	1 gram	3 grams

Percentage of U.S. Recommended Daily Allowance (U.S. RDA) for adults and children over 12 years

	Per Meal	Per Day (3 Meals)
Protein	25	75
Vitamin A	33⅓	100
Vitamin C	33⅓	100
Thiamine	33⅓	100
Riboflavin	33⅓	100
Niacin	33⅓	100
Calcium	33⅓	100
Iron	33⅓	100
Vitamin D	33⅓	100
Vitamin E	33⅓	100
Vitamin B6	33⅓	100
Folic Acid	33⅓	100
Vitamin B12	33⅓	100
Phosphorus	33⅓	100
Iodine	33⅓	100
Magnesium	33⅓	100
Zinc	33⅓	100
Copper	33⅓	100
Biotin	33⅓	100
Pantothenic Acid	33⅓	100
Vitamin K*	22.3 mcg	67 mcg
Sodium* (1490 mg/100 g)	500 mg	1500 mg**
Potassium*	670 mg	2010 mg**
Manganese*	1.3 mg	4 mg**
Chloride*	600 mg	1800 mg**
Chromium*	20 mcg	60 mcg**
Selenium*	20 mcg	60 mcg**
Molybdenum*	50 mcg	150 mcg**

*U.S. RDA has not been established.
**The Food and Nutrition Board of the National Research Council recommends these quantities of these essential trace minerals as being within the range required in the diet of an adult.

BIBLIOGRAPHY

Published studies relating to the development of Cambridge Diet by Dr. Alan N. Howard and coworkers at the Department of Medicine, University of Cambridge, Addenbrooke's Hospital, Hills Road, Cambridge CB2 2QQ, England, and the West Middlesex Hospital, London.

1. "Dietary treatment of obesity." Howard, A.N. (1975). *Obesity: Its Pathogenesis and Management.* Edited by Silverstone, T. Medical and Technical Publishing Co. Ltd. pp. 123–154.

2. "The treatment of obesity by starvation and semi-starvation." Howard, A.N. (1979). *The Treatment of Obesity.* Edited by Munro, J.F. MTP Press, Ltd., England. pp. 139–164.

3. "Possible complications of long-term dietary treatment of obesity." Howard, A.N. (1979). *Proceedings of Serono Symposium.* Edited by Mancini, M., Lewis, B., and Contaldo, F. Academic Press, London, pp. 349–363.

4. "The long term treatment of obesity by low calorie semi-synthetic formula diets." Howard, A.N. and McLean Baird, I. (1972). IX International Congress of Nutrition, Mexico.

5. "The treatment of obesity by low calorie diets containing amino acids." Howard, A.N. and McLean Baird, I. (1973). *Nutrition and Dietetics.*

6. "Clinical and metabolic studies of chemically defined diets in the management of obesity." McLean Baird, I., Parsons, R.L. and Howard, A.N. *Metabolism* 23 (1974): 645–657.

7. "The treatment of obesity by low calorie semi-synthetic diets." Howard, A.N. and McLean Biard, I. (1974). *Recent Advances in Obesity Research: 1.* Edited by Howard A.N. Newman Publishing Ltd. pp. 270–273.

8. "Very low calorie semisynthetic diets in the treatment of obesity." An inpatient/outpatient study. Howard, A.N. and McLean Baird, I. *Nutr. Metab.* 21 (1977): 59–61.

9. "A long-term evaluation of very low calorie semisynthetic diets: an inpatient/outpatient study with egg albumin as the protein source." Howard, A.N. and McLean Baird, I. *International Journal of Obesity* 1 (1977): 63–78.

10. "A double-blind trial of mazindol using a very low calorie formula diet." McLean Baird, I. and Howard, A.N. *International Journal of Obesity* 1 (1977): 271–278.

11. "The treatment of obesity with a very low calorie liquid-formula diet: an inpatient/outpatient comparison using skimmed-milk protein as the chief protein source." Howard, A.N. Grant, A., Edwards, O., Littlewood, E.R. and McLean Baird, I. *International Journal of Obesity* 2 (1978): 321–332.

12. "Thyroid metabolism in obese subjects after a very low calorie diet." Howard, A.N., Grant, A., Challand, G., Wraight, E.P. and Edwards, O. (1977). Second International Congress on Obesity.

13. "Faecal transit time and nitrogen balance in patients receiving a new low calorie formula diet." McLean Baird, E., Littlewood, I.R. and Howard, A.N. (1977). Second International Congress on Obesity.

14. "Thyroid metabolism in obese subjects after a very low calorie diet." Howard, A.N., Grant, A., Challand, G., Wraight, E.P. and Edwards, O. *International Journal of Obesity* 2 (1978): 391.

15. "Thyroidal hormone metabolism in obesity during semi-starvation." Grant, A.M., Edwards, O.M., Howard, A.N., Challand, G., Wraight, E.P. and Mills, I.H. *Clinical Endocrinology* 9 (1978): 227–231.

16. "Treatment of obesity with triiodothyronine and a very-low-calorie liquid formula diet." Moore, R., Grant, A.M., Howard, A.N. and Mills, I.H. (1980). *The Lancet* (Feb. 2, 1980), pp. 223–226.

17. "Safety of very low calorie diets." McLean Baird, I., Littlewood, E.R. and Howard, A.N. *International Journal of Obesity* 3 (1979): 399.

18. "The historical development, efficacy and safety of very low calorie diets." Howard, A.N. *International Journal of Obesity* 5 (1981): 195–208.

19. "Low-dose mianserin as adjuvant therapy in obese patients treated by a very low calorie diet." Cook, R.F., Howard, A.N., and Mills, I.H. *International Journal of Obesity* 5 (1981): 267–272.

20. "Changes in thyroid hormone levels, kinetics and cell receptors in obese patients treated with T_3 and a very low calorie formula diet." Moore, R., Grant, A.M., Howard, A.N., Mehrishi, J.N., and Mills, I.H. (1981). In: *Recent Advances in Clinical Nutrition*. J. Libbey & Co., Ltd., London.

21. "Physiopathology of protein metabolism in relation to very low calorie regimens." Howard, A.N., and McLean Baird, I. (1981). In: *Recent Advances in Obesity Research: III*. John Libbey & Co., Ltd., London.

22. "Low calorie formula diets — are they safe?" McLean Baird, I. *International Journal of Obesity* 5 (1981): 249–256.

23. "The role of T_3 and its receptor in efficient metabolisers receiving very low calorie diets." Moore, R., Mehrishi, J.N., Verdoorn, C. and Mills, I.H. *International Journal of Obesity* 5 (1981): 283–296.

Studies on Cambridge Diet at other centers

24. "Report of a comparative study: a new very low calorie formula diet versus a conventional diet in the treatment of obesity." Shapiro, H.J. *International Journal of Obesity* 2 (1978): 392.

25. "Serum Thyroid Hormone Concentrations During Prolonged Reduction of Dietary Intake." Visser, T. J, Lamberts, S.W.J., Wilson, J.H.P., Docter, R. and Hennemann, G. (1978). *Metabolism,* Vol. 27, No. 4, pp. 405–409.

26. "Nitrogen balance in obese patients receiving a very low calorie liquid formula diet." Wilson, J.H.P. and Lamberts, S.W.J. *American Journal of Clinical Nutrition* 32 (1979): pp. 1612–1616.

27. "The influence of caloric restrictions on serum prolactin." Lamberts, S.W.J., Visser, T.J., and Wilson, J.H.P. *International Journal of Obesity* 3 (1979): 75–81.

28. "The effect of triiodothyronine on weight loss and nitrogen balance of obese patients on a very low calorie liquid formula diet." Wilson, J.H.P. and Lamberts, W.J. *International Journal of Obesity* 5 (1981): 279–282.

29. "The effect of obesity and drastic caloric restriction on serum prolactin and thyroid stimulating hormone." Wilson, J.H.P. and Lamberts, S.W.J. *International Journal of Obesity* 5 (1981): 275–278.

30. "Outpatient treatment of obesity with a very low calorie formula diet." Hickey, N., Daly, L., Bourke, G. and Mulcahy, R. *International Journal of Obesity* 5 (1981): 227–230.

31. "The effect of a very low calorie diet with and without chronic exercise on thyroid and sex hormones, plasma proteins, oxygen uptake, insulin and c peptide concentrations in obese women." Krotkiewski, M., Toss, L., Björntorp, P. and Holm, G. *International Journal of Obesity* 5 (1981): 287–293.

32. "A very low calorie formula diet (Cambridge Diet) for the treatment of diabetic-obese patients." DiBiase, G., Mattioli, P.L., Contaldo, F. and Mancini, M. *International Journal of Obesity* 5 (1981): 319–324.